"I've known Benjamin for m̠
to a competent adult. I knov
neurotypical world. He write
spectrum face, and by bring.
through his writing he offers hope to those who are raising a child with
autism. He has a passion and a vision to make a difference in people's
lives."

Dr. Mary MacDonald
Developmental Pediatrician

"Benjamin Collier writes from personal experience. As one who has
lived his life seeing the world through the eyes of autism, he is more
than qualified to share the struggles and triumphs. Benjamin has learned
how to laugh--at himself and with others. He has learned the art of
expression and now offers his knowlege to those who are facing the same
trials. Benjamin's book is filled with humour and heartbreak and leaves
the reader cheering."

Donna Fawcett
award winning novelist and
author of the writing tutorial
Duke the Chihuahua Writes!

"Ben Collier writes with a clear, concise and engaging voice. His wit and
insight keep me coming back to his work."

C.L. Dyck, freelance writer and editor

An Inside Look at Autism and Asperger's Syndrome

MY LIFE A.S. IS

Benjamin T. Collier

MY LIFE A.S. IS
Copyright © 2013 by Benjamin T. Collier

Scriptures taken from the Holy Bible, New International Version®, NIV®. Copyright © 1973, 1978, 1984, 2011 by Biblica, Inc.™ Used by permission of Zondervan. All rights reserved worldwide. www.zondervan.com. The "NIV" and "New International Version" are trademarks registered in the United States Patent and Trademark Office by Biblica, Inc.™

ISBN: 978-1-77069-778-2

Word Alive Press
131 Cordite Road, Winnipeg, MB R3W 1S1
www.wordalivepress.ca

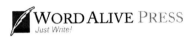

Library and Archives Canada Cataloguing in Publication
Collier, Benjamin T., 1983-
    My life A.S. is : an inside look at autism and Asperger's syndrome / Benjamin T. Collier.
ISBN 978-1-77069-778-2
    1. Collier, Benjamin T., 1983-. 2. Asperger's syndrome--Patients--Biography. 3. Asperger's syndrome. I. Title.
RC553.A88C65 2013   616.85'8820092   C2012-907756-9

"If you was hit by a truck and you were lyin' out in that gutter dyin' and you had time to sing one song, one song people would remember before you're dirt, one song that would let God know what you felt about your time here on earth, one song that would sum you up—you tellin' me that's the song you'd sing? That same Jimmie Davis tune we hear on the radio all day? About your 'peace within' and how 'it's real' and how you're 'gonna shout it'? Or would you sing somethin' different? Somethin' real, somethin' you felt? Because I'm tellin' you right now, that's the kind of song people want to hear. That's the kind of song that truly saves people."

—*Walk the Line*

This is good, and pleases God our Savior, who wants all men to be saved and to come to a knowledge of the truth.

—1 Timothy 2:3–4

TABLE OF CONTENTS

ACKNOWLEDGEMENTS

I wish to thank Anna, my little big sister, for always encouraging me in my ways; Karen, my princess, for reaching into my world when nobody else knew how; Dad, for working so hard to provide for all of us; and Mum, for being my rock, my encouragement, my strength, and my hope, for fighting for me and *growling* at the masses when they attacked, for being the hippest mom on the planet, and for always encouraging me to be myself.

I also thank Shanks, just for being you—because of you I'm not alone in this world; Dr. Mary MacDonald, for helping those around me understand my world; the Alpha Ministry team, for some of the best and most powerful experiences of my life; and the Word Guild, for giving me so much love and encouragement to complete this book.

I must also thank the Father, full of so much imagination and creativity. Thank you for letting me see the world, and for giving me the gifts to interact with it. And to the Son; I will never realize how much you did for me, but I'm enjoying the journey. Thank you for showing me the way, for calling me "friend." Thank you to the Holy Spirit, for helping me come so far. I know I would not be the same without you. Thank you for enabling me to see other people, to see the worlds within them, and to link our worlds together.

TO MY NIECE AND NEPHEWS

Josiah, thank you for making me like kids again. Because of you, I remember everything God uses to bring joy into my life. You are so strong. You've inherited so much Spirit. I see in you the kind of wisdom-beyond-your-years that people saw in me at your age, and you handle it like a pro.

Caleb, I'm sorry I didn't get to know you. I didn't dote on you while you were in the womb, figuring I'd have plenty of time after you were born. I won't make that mistake again. I hope God is preparing you for the torrent of hugs you'll get when we all finally see you.

Kara, Little Princess, you are both beautiful and smart. That is a rare combination, but I see these in you along with a gracious heart that melds it all together. You are not afraid to be yourself. I love watching the lady you are growing up to be.

Elijah Thunder, your birth was difficult—like mine. You had many opportunities to leave this world, but you refused. You're a fighter. No one can take that away from you. I know this world is challenging, but keep your eyes on God. He has plans for you and will fight alongside you.

Nate, you make everybody smile. You have no idea how remarkable that gift is. You've had such a powerful ministry already. I love your creativity. I see many of my own quirks in you. Always be yourself. I'm looking forward to seeing what God will do with you.

I t was a scary year when I sat down to write this. The toughest I'd been through by far. My place in the world never seemed so uncertain. It's not so much a question of "Why am I here?" so much as "Why did God take a person like me and put me in a world like this?" This world and I don't get along. We can't see eye to eye. The rules of this world are a foreign language to me. We're not compatible.

Why stress over it?

Aside from the initial frustration of not seeing God's logic in putting me here, there is also the deep need we all feel—the need to justify our existence. If we don't do something productive with our lives, how can we look our Creator in the face? We want to be able to say to Him, "You did not make me in vain. I was not a waste of matter."

But when I really think about it, if I was created by an intelligent God then I'm not my own creation. Therefore it is not my place to justify my existence—it's His. I am His work. For some reason, He saw fit to make me. He took pleasure in the fine details of my personality, my intellect, my random humour, my sense of honesty.

But then He put me here.

Why?

I know I'm not the only one asking such questions. Asperger's Syndrome (A.S.) and related conditions on the Autism Spectrum Disorder (A.S.D.) are popping up in greater numbers than ever before, affecting one in every hundred fifty at the time of this writing. Still, most of the public is in the dark when it comes to understanding such people, since so few of them can actually describe what they're going through. Many parents of A.S.D. children are left completely unaware of what they can do to bridge the gap between their world and the so distant inner world of their child.

As someone who was severely autistic as a young child, and who grew up with A.S., this book is my attempt to describe what it was like to be in my world, and what it's like for me to live in your world now.

Although this book is about me, it's impossible to talk about myself in depth without mentioning God. He is such a major, out-in-the-open part of my life that He pervades everything in it. I know I wouldn't have developed this far without His help. I was completely lost in my own world. Most of the time I wasn't even aware that another world existed. I couldn't have come out of it on my own. It took an outside force, a force beyond myself, to help me cross between worlds.

I've been working on this book for a number of years. Even now, as I go back to add little bits of information, I'm encouraged to see how far I've come in just a few years. The changes in feelings and perceptions I otherwise wouldn't have noticed are more apparent to me now that I've gone back and read what I was going through before. God has been at work in me.

I spent the first twenty-three years of my life being secretive about my condition. My code of honesty required me to say I had Asperger's if anyone asked, but I never volunteered the information and it rarely came up in conversation. It's not a physically recognizable condition, as opposed to Down's Syndrome; people with A.S.D. typically just appear to be distant-minded.

I've always wanted people to get to know me personally before discovering my "specialness." I don't want people to treat me differently because of my "handicap." I have always needed to know I could function and be accepted in the world before letting anyone know about my condition.

That time is passed. I'm tired of being misunderstood and misjudged, which I think we can all relate to. Hopefully my full disclosure will help people to understand the depth of anxiety and frustration people with Asperger's typically experience.

I find it difficult to pinpoint certain areas where my thought processes differ from those of others. Having never been without A.S., I have no point of reference for what an average person thinks and feels. Perhaps if someone came out with a book explaining the functionality of the typical human being I would have a better perspective on what the differences are, but I suppose a book like that wouldn't sell.

I think it's important to note that my observations in this book come from my own experiences and may not reflect people with Asperger's as a whole—nor will everyone with Asperger's share the same traits—yet some similarities are to be expected. I hope this book helps to clarify which traits are commonly shared between people with A.S. and which are due to individual uniqueness.

Autism and Asperger's are definitely linked, as I seemed to "upgrade" from one to the other as I got older. Asperger's is considered the more "normal" of the two, sometimes called "high-functioning autism," though a general disdain for social conduct exists in both. Both also contain heavy doses of Attention Deficit Disorder (A.D.D.) and its hyperactive cousin, A.D.H.D. Although some may view Asperger's and autism as separate conditions, I see Asperger's as resting somewhere on the Autism Spectrum, even though having Asperger's and having autism feel like two different things. That's why I'll make references to myself as having both conditions; over the course of my life, I have switched from one condition to the other.

Many aspects of my mentality can lead one to conclude that I'm a complete jerk by nature. That conclusion would not be entirely unfounded. I have observed that when I don't make a conscious effort to be decent, my natural personality contains a lot of cynicism, anger, impatience, and bigotry—to name a few of my failings. By opening up about these things, I'm not condoning or excusing them; I'm simply acknowledging that I struggle with them.

Know that the progress I've made in moving away from complete jerkness has been a joint effort between myself and God, who has been working to clean the crap out of my heart since I was five. There is still much work to do!

MY PERSPECTIVE

I believe the first thing I said when I was told I had Asperger's was, "I have ass burgers?"

All my life, I've been proud of my autism as the thing that makes me unique. But I realize now that this line of reasoning is flawed, because my autism is not my identity. It's not a part of my core being. It couldn't have been responsible for my sense of humour, my likes or dislikes, or my relationship with God. However, I believe autism has provided the necessary environment for me to embrace myself as fully as I have. It has removed the need to "fit in," which most people do by suppressing anything about themselves they don't see in others.

I believe that God has made each of us unique, but most of us are uncomfortable with being different from the crowd. Many of us who do want to be unique have a hard time pinpointing what it is that makes us stand out. I have a blessing most people don't, which is an identified and perfect excuse to be unique.

One extreme approach to autism is to view it as a disease of which we need to be cured. I understand how difficult it can be to live with, and I understand that not everyone has it as mildly as I do. But many parents have come to the same conclusion that my mother did—that it isn't a disease, but a part of who we are meant to be.

Some parents have taken the other extreme and feel that autism is an inseparable part of their child's person. They don't want a cure for autism because they feel their child wouldn't be themself if they were "cured." This borders on what I call the "Wolverine Complex" (see the appendix).

Still others have said that autism is part of the continuing evolution of humanity, perhaps the early stages of the next big leap, or a separate line of evolution that would produce a race of cousins to "normal" humanity.

I don't feel that any extreme view is healthy.

Of course, everyone should be proud of who they are, as God made them to be. The problem is that most of us don't differentiate between *who we are* and *what we have*. At present, we don't know how much of autism is genetic and how much is personality. If I didn't have autism, would I still be myself? Of course I would! But the truth is that even without autism, I would still be quiet, intelligent, deep, honest, and funny—because those are all parts of who I am. Thus, autism may actually be the "condition" that best suits my personality.

THE PERSPECTIVE OF OTHERS

Most people respond to me with curiosity. Some people seem afraid of me, particularly single women (I probably stare too much). Very few flat-out hate me, but when they do it's usually due to a misunderstanding, like when people meet me only briefly and don't understand my quirks.

I have noticed that people who are in great pain fall into two groups: those who are attracted to me and those who hate me. Most people in pain perceive that I'm sensitive and patient enough to talk to them one-on-one and listen without passing judgement. Others see me as too perfect and refuse to accept that a person like me could exist, or they see me as self-righteous and superficial. Or perhaps a complicated mixture of both.

Indeed, I do often come across as innocent and naïve, and to some extent I am, but I'm not innocent to the extent that people seem to think. I've lived a very sheltered life, distant from the most common temptations, but I know that when given the opportunity to sin I'm just as attracted to it as everyone else.

Even many high-functioning autistics may come across as self-centred. This is to be expected, since we've spent much of our lives in our own world, where we don't have anyone else to think about. That was our introduction to life. Even if we are aware of other people now, we have to contend with an old, built-in worldview and all the habits that go with it.

When people make an effort to get to know me, they usually find me refreshing and unique.

A problem I keep running into, though, is that people want to change me, to make me more like them. Even though people appreciate me for my uniqueness, they still want to pull me into being one of the crowd. People still can't recognize that some of us are called by God into a different kind of life.

I understand that some things are standard for everyone, but as an autistic, I'm not standard. I excel in some areas and fall short in others. With no guidelines on the typical life of an autistic, I had no starting ground of what should and shouldn't be expected of me. And developing from severe autism to high-functioning autism meant I wasn't sure how close to standard I had become, and how much I still lacked.

This created a lot of anxiety for me as I entered early adulthood. I'd heard so much about what I ought to do that I could no longer distinguish between what other people expected of me, what I expected of myself, and what God expected of me.

HOW IT FEELS

One of the reasons deep autistics don't communicate is because they don't see a need to. When there's a problem, they believe that everyone already knows what the problem is. The view of an autistic is that everyone knows what they know, as if they are of a single consciousness. No, an autistic cannot read minds, but they aren't even aware that there is any mind other than their own. Therefore, when there is a problem, everyone should know the problem and try to solve it. This is why it's so frustrating that the problem isn't already solved.

As a child, I remember wondering if my bad thoughts ever bothered the people around me. But I think that was already an improvement. Before that, I wouldn't have considered that anyone even had feelings other than my own.

As a child, it was like my presence was hooked up to a megaphone—my awareness of my own presence was so "loud" that I wasn't aware of the presence of anyone else. I felt out in the open, vulnerable, under constant observation. Even now, when I'm out in public I feel like I'm the centre of attention. I know that I'm not, but I always feel like I'm under surveillance. And it's not just God giving me that feeling, because it isn't always a peaceful, freeing feeling.

I had a constant mental image in my head of what I looked like as I did something, as if I watched my every move through my own camera just off to the side. Now, the mental camera is only on at specific times, and I'm aware of the inaccuracy of my mental image of myself, but as a child I could picture exactly how I looked as I did everything.

Oddly enough, I actually feel more disconnected from my environment when I'm on my own, meaning when I'm not with someone I know. I could be in a shopping mall full of people and feel completely disconnected. But if I'm walking with someone I know, I tend to feel part of my environment.

You would think that having to act on my own would make me more alert. Instead it just makes me more focused on my task, and even less aware of my surroundings. This isn't extreme, of course; I don't crash into things when I'm on my own, but I don't feel that I'm a part of my environment.

Though I've felt more connected when walking through my backyard lately, that same yard used to be a weird place for me. It's a forested area next to the Ganaraska River. I spent so much time indoors, surrounded by manmade things, that whenever I went outside, surrounded by God's handiwork, God had so much to say to me through nature. Too much. Going outside was like being bombarded by a thousand words at once.

Over time, I walked through my backyard frequently enough that the initial torrent of information calmed to a relaxing and refreshing stream. I could go outside and look forward to the time spent with God's creation, listening to what He had to say through His work. It became fertile ground for inspiration and deep spiritual discussions.

When I walk into a room full of people, even if it's a room I spend a lot of time in, the mass of moving, thinking, changing people disorients me completely to the point that I may appear wasted. More than once, I've been mistaken for a junkie because of my complexion, long hair, and distant attitude. I also have an awesome pair of shades that make me look like John Lennon.

Autistic children usually progress at a normal pace for the first fifteen months and then suddenly shift into reverse, losing any and all communication skills they may have learned to that point. This fuels the theory that children aren't born with it but that it's caused by something like a vaccine. My mother testifies that my non-development was constant since birth; I didn't follow the usual developmental route before reverting; I never developed normally to begin with, until my turnaround at the age of five. I don't know if my case is unique.

CHAPTER ONE

Unique Features

SENSITIVITY

Hypersensitivity, in one or all categories, is common for autistics, even while they may be unresponsive to other senses. In my case, I'm oversensitive to taste and sound, and under sensitive to touch. Autistics generally have an all-around intolerance of loud noises which would seem soft to the average person.

My ears struggle to take in loud, reverberating sounds. It's easier outdoors, but even outdoors there are some noises, such as megaphones, that I can't handle. It's like my ear nerves work too slowly to process all the sound waves bouncing off my eardrums. The result is feeling overwhelmed, like the walls of my ears are going to collapse from the bombardment, sending vibrations directly into my head. It's a scary feeling.

I have little perception of the volume of my own voice and typically have a very monotonous, Johnny Cash kind of tone. I don't perceive how loud or quiet I am. I often mumble. When people tell me I need to speak up, which happens often, I either mumble a bit more or I have to shout; I have no in-between. It's like everyone's voice has forty levels of volume, and most people have a button for each volume. But I have only two buttons—quiet and loud. My quiet button ranges from volumes one to ten and is usually set at five, but my loud button moves randomly from anywhere between volumes eleven and forty. When I press the loud button, I have no idea what volume my voice will be, so I press that button reluctantly.

It's very difficult to be in a crowd of people, especially in a tight space. This is one reason why I socialize much more easily one-on-one than I do in group settings.

When I read that many Asperger's people have gastrointestinal disorders due to selective eating habits, I recognized my own eating issues right away. When I then read that selective eating could be due to oversensitive taste, I almost laughed.

Most of us can force ourselves to finish a meal, even if it tastes bad. For me, however, a poor meal doesn't just taste bad—it tastes downright evil! I've caught myself breathing abnormally while trying to chew something. I wasn't even aware I was doing it until the noise became loud enough. It was my natural response to feeling what was in my mouth. I thought to myself, "It's just food. Get over it!"

This is the reason I dread having dinner at a friend's house. My mother is used to me, but I'm very bad at hiding my true feelings when I'm eating something. Even when I determine to say nothing, I have very little control over my facial responses. If you ever invite me over to your house, I would advise takeout.

Touch may be another sense that's higher in some areas and lower in others. I have slightly above average tolerance to pain. I normally don't realize when I'm too hot unless someone asks me if I'm hot, and of course I say "Yes." It usually takes someone else to point out the temperature before I notice how I feel.

When I was five, I came home from school once to find my sister Karen freaking out because of a massive bloodstain on my back, as if I'd been shot there. Apparently while playing, I had fallen onto a pointy rock and hadn't noticed.

A lot of nurses think I'm afraid of needles, but taking shots doesn't bother me; it's blood tests that bother me. It's not the feeling of the needle but the awareness that my lifeblood is being drained from my body. I'm unable to process it without growing faint.

This may be hemophobia, but I think there's more to it than that. I seem to grow faint whenever I suffer an injury I don't understand. I've spent several minutes over the bathroom sink watching my own blood drain from my nose without being scared. I've dealt with nosebleeds enough times to know I'll be okay. But something as simple as a bruise under my fingernail can cause queasiness, simply because I don't understand the injury.

I have handled blood tests better in recent years. Previously I went to great lengths to be as unaware of what was going on as possible, looking away from the needle, refusing to see my blood. But I would still grow faint when I saw the patch on my arm. The problem was that I had to come to terms with what had happened to me, realize it was okay, and move on.

My strategy in recent years has been to lie down and look away as the blood is being taken, then look at the patch on my arm for a long time, thinking about this horrible thing that was done to my body.

The jerks! What gives them the right? Look what they've done to my arm!

Then I'm okay.

The fact is, whether I know intellectually that it's okay or not, my body really doesn't like having blood taken. It's foundationally opposed to it. I have to let my body know that I understand, that I feel it, and that it hurt me. Only then can I tell myself, and my body, that I endured the ordeal.

It's also a matter of focus. A number of times while in the middle of a task, I've noticed an injury and continued to work with no problem. As long as I have something to do, I'm okay. But if the task is finished and my injury remains, I may go into brief, mild shock. Fortunately, it doesn't last long, because I've already had it long enough to know that I'll be okay.

When I had my wisdom teeth removed, it was a lot easier than everyone told me it would be. My drug intake was low. After one dose, I stopped taking the extra-strength painkillers, figuring I didn't need them. Besides, I was much more comfortable with pain than disorientation. I stuck with milder painkillers.

Immediately after the surgery—or rather, the first thing I remember after surgery—was waking up in the recovery room. My mouth was full of paper to soak up the blood. I was told not to speak. I observed my left hand and saw the bandages where the IV had been removed. That IV injury was the first thing I had to deal with. My mouth was still numb and I couldn't see it, but the IV bandage I could plainly see. I wrote on a notepad that before I got up I needed a moment to look at my hand and process what had happened.

When I got home, I was given the task of removing the paper from my mouth, with my head over the sink. So much blood poured out of my mouth that it was like watching *Mortal Kombat*. I laughed, to my mother's surprise and relief. I put some new paper in my mouth and moved on—I was perfectly fine, if maybe a little high.

I have other areas of sensitivity. For example, I've always regarded feet as something personal. As a child, I considered them almost a private part. I didn't like being barefoot, and I didn't like seeing other people's bare feet. And the worst thing possible was for someone else's bare feet to touch mine—that felt like violation.

One day when my mom took me to the beach, she told me I had to take my shoes and socks off. I refused. It became a power struggle, and she pulled off my shoes and socks herself. I ran away, curled up in a ball, and buried my feet in the sand. I stayed like that for a long time before I was comfortable to move again.

ODD WRITING

When I was first being taught to handwrite, like everyone else I was taught to draw letters from the top down. For some reason, I couldn't do this the way school wanted me to, because I always drew through the line that was supposed to mark the bottom. I could only draw a proper letter if I started at the bottom, on the line, and drew upward. So that's how I learned to write, and it's still how I write today.

My uncle saw me write recently and noted how freaky it was. "It's as if you start where you're supposed to finish and the words just appear!"

My childhood difficulty with differentiating between letters led me to focus on uppercase for years. Even today, my natural handwriting is in all caps. I passed English, so I'm fully capable of writing upper and lowercase when there's a need for formality, but it slows me down. Hence, all the notes lying around the house are in all caps.

I never took to fancy handwriting, the kind where all the letters have to connect. I'm sure there are some people who are able to write in that style fluently, but I haven't read anything by them. Every time I come across that kind of writing it's a garbled, lazy mess and I have to ask someone else to read it for me; quite often, though, I can't find anyone who can.

For both reading and writing I much prefer print style.

SELECTIVE TIDYNESS

The most accurate phrase, if you were to see my room, would be "selective tidyness." Some things are perfectly neat and organized while others are dropped randomly in the relative vicinity of where they should be. Still others have no place at all—yet may appear tidy wherever they happen to be.

The organizational system of my stuff is *practical*. Items are placed (tidely or otherwise) in proximity to my chair in the order of how frequently they're used. When I'm in a Pokémon mood, my Pokémon cards will be closer to my chair than my video game magazines.

As for which stuff is made tidy and which is left untidy, I think it a matter of chance based on whatever happens to be in view when the urge to clean strikes me, which doesn't happen often.

MY IMAGINATION

I have a very effective, natural anti-boredom mechanism. When I get bored, I use my imagination. It tends to work best if I'm in a particular mood—a *Star Wars* mood, a Terminator mood, a Jedi mood, etc. (Yes, there's a difference between a *Star Wars* mood and a Jedi mood... a *big* difference). When I'm in a particular mood, my thoughts are focused. This allows me to obsess over a single subject for an extended length of time. It's actually strenuous when I'm not in a particular mood, because my thoughts will flit from one subject to another; I can't get into deep thought when I do that, and deep thought is where I find real significance.

My imagination allowed me to survive a childhood of following my mother around shopping malls, working at my sister's clothing store, and spending seven years as an extra in film and television—which, by the way, isn't very exciting.

Of course, in my earliest years my imagination was the barrier keeping me from the rest of the world, but once I learned how to step in and out of my imagination, I was able to use it to my advantage.

Revisiting some of the places I knew as a child, I can walk into one and remember a video game I invented while waiting there. I recently followed my mom into a women's clothing store and remembered inventing a fighting game consisting entirely of dead people—skeletons, zombies, snake skeletons, and six-armed skeletons. (It was during my nasty-things-are-cool phase, which lasted until I was fifteen.)

Most people visit a place from their childhood and can tell you exactly what they used to do there. I visit a place from my childhood and can tell you what I used to think about. "That corridor reminded me of that scene from *The Labyrinth*." "Over here I imagined the Shredder on a pirate ship over the Sarlacc Pit." "This is where I imagined what it looked like when God was putting people together." And this is what makes the place familiar and comforting.

I don't recall ever having an imaginary friend, but my mother says I used to imagine the Ninja Turtles coming with me to school every day in Grade One, which made it difficult for me to pay attention in class. The problem was resolved when she told me the Turtles had to go to Turtle School instead.

I do recall occasionally trying to play with imaginary friends, but it never worked out; by the time it occurred to me that I could do that, I was fully aware that these characters were fictional. Knowing that something was imaginary didn't make it any less vivid, but certainly less social.

I've enjoyed countless hours in my own world, even when I was aware that it wasn't the *real* world. I've endured hours of waiting around in boring places either on set or going shopping with someone. I survived because of my ability to go somewhere else in my mind.

I do have mental conversations with myself—but I don't know anybody who doesn't. One thing about my mental conversations is that

I use them to debate with myself. I'm able to argue, even sympathize with, a side that I disagree with. Why? Because my beliefs are constantly under attack and sometimes the other side of an argument has good points. It's important for me to be able to response to tough questions, especially regarding my faith, responses that will draw people closer to God rather than push them away. In the heat of an argument, I don't always have the grace I should to represent the word of God, so it's important to think these debates through in a setting where I can take my time and be calm with my responses.

There may be a number of reasons why I'm able to sympathize with sides I disagree with. I hear countless varying opinions and personal stories when I watch TV or read books. Most important is the ability to recognize that these aren't just opinions contradicting my beliefs; they're coming from real people, many of them in real pain. I need to make their pain my own before I can find the words to bring them to the truth I know.

THOUGHT TRAVEL

How do I explain the way my thought process works?

It's like the human brain is the garage for a delivery service, and every package is a thought, and each part of the brain is a different terrain vehicle. My brain has to deliver a thought across a desert wilderness, only my desert jeep won't start, so I'm stuck with a snowmobile. Not only that but the snowmobile already has packages of its own to deliver, so it has to work double-time.

The package still gets there, but it's slower, and because it's a different vehicle it can't take the same routes, resulting in a different journey. So whenever someone asks me a question, my thought takes longer to process, and often provides a different perspective because it had to take a different path.

Ironically, the side of my brain that doesn't operate right is the logic side, yet people find me to be very logical—almost Spock-like when you add the lack of emotion on my face.

The truth is that I've come to some very wise decisions through purely creative means. In certain moments, I'll have a sense of the right thing to do, but in the moment I have no idea why it's the right thing to do. It isn't until after the situation is over, and I have time to think about it, that I realize why it was right.

My current theory is that this sense of right came from observing appropriate behaviour in movies like *The Lord of the Rings* and shows like *Star Trek: The Next Generation*—anything in which you have people of rank talking to their superiors and subordinates with due respect and propriety. As long as an atmosphere of mutual respect is kept, a respect that is true and not superficial, it will have the right effect on the people watching it.

See, I may not know logically why someone does things a certain way, but I can learn their way through observance nonetheless.

One example of using creativity to reach a logical conclusion may be the use of allegory. However, most autistics are unable to extrapolate connections between one thing and another—it's too abstract. I had that problem as a child as well. I don't know how I grew out of it, but now I'm able to see connections between practically everything.

I can see how Bible verses from millennia ago mirror events happening today, both around the world and in my own life. I see Jesus parallels in stories that I'm pretty sure were unintentional. For example, in *The Chronicles of Riddick*. The character of Riddick lets himself get captured and sent to prison to rescue a friend of his (like Jesus letting himself get captured and die on the cross to save *his* friends). During the escape, everyone has to get from the prison to the hanger, across miles of desert, before the sun rises, so Riddick says, "There's gonna be one speed—mine. If you can't keep up, don't step up—you'll just die." When God brought the Israelites out of captivity in Egypt, He gave them the Ten Commandments and the rest of the Old Testament laws. Those laws were the standard of perfection. If you wanted to earn your place in heaven, you had to follow those laws by the letter... laws that only Jesus ever successfully fulfilled. In other words, God demands one "speed" from his followers.

Riddick's friend tries to keep up with him but falls behind (missing the mark—the definition of sin), but Riddick went back and rescued her anyway, suffering the punishing heat of the sun, a penalty reserved for another.

I see parallels in the most unlikely places, which is probably why I'm geared to write allegorical stories. I've even concluded that my gift for finding parallels is the reason my middle name is Thomas (meaning "Twin").

Time Perception

I tend to get lost in activities and lose track of time. That's probably normal, but I also seem to blend my entire history into parallel timelines when I think about the past. For example, I'll remember something from years ago as if it were months or weeks ago. I still regard the nineties as "just before now" and kind of clump all of the 2000 years into a short period of time. And it's hard to picture something I did in my childhood or teen years as being "a long time ago." For that reason, I'm still embarrassed and ashamed of many of the mistakes I made in those years, as if I haven't matured since then.

Teamwork

It's common for me to have difficulty operating in a team. Perhaps that's because I can't give my attention to the needs of each individual while at the same time paying attention to the needs of the group as a whole. It's much easier to focus on what I can do, and just do it.

The main reason teamwork is so difficult for an autistic person isn't incompetence. It's that autistics are specialists. We're extraordinarily gifted in specific areas, and lacking in others. Society says that everyone should be the same, and perform the same in every aspect of life. If you're a specialist, then you're an outcast, because although you excel in one area, you fail in all other "essential" areas.

Most teams are organized with the assumption that everyone should perform the same task with the same level of skill as everybody else. Instead of each player being assigned according to their strengths, to the specific tasks they do best, everyone is lumped together as a collective whole, each one expected to perform as efficiently as everyone else at the same task. This results in the *weakest link* mentality, and with this kind of organization the weakest link is always the specialist.

I personally like the idea of teamwork. I like seeing how people with different strengths can come together to accomplish a common goal. Unfortunately, some team leaders don't bother to organize players according to their strengths; it's much easier to just tell them all to do the same thing and cut out anyone who doesn't perform well.

I never hear or remember everything I'm supposed to when I'm in a meeting. It helps a lot to have another person to help me to review what was said. It isn't that I don't care what other people say; it's that I care so much about a particular thing the person has said that I don't hear what they say afterward. I *am* listening, but I'm still listening to what they said half an hour ago.

Part of the reason for that is that I process information at a slower rate than most, which is a result of autism. That said, thanks to John Eldredge in his book *Wild at Heart*, I'm being led to believe that A.D.D. in most cases isn't so much a disorder as a personality trait. One of his points is that A.D.D. is far more common in males than females, to the extent that varying degrees of it can be found in almost every male if you observe closely enough. But because girls are more patient and better listeners in the classroom, they're held up as standard students. Anyone who doesn't learn as fast as a typical girl is therefore labelled with a disorder and must be treated for it until they're able to think like a girl.

SPEAKING

I'm told that I was nonverbal up until the age of four. I knew very few words and I didn't know how to use them. At the age of four, I was old enough to understand that Jesus was my Saviour, though I didn't understand how until later. That was the time I officially gave myself to God. After that, I started communicating with words, properly. I didn't shut up until I was thirteen.

ECHOLALIA

When I was first learning to talk, I couldn't originate my own words. Instead I imitated what I heard on movies and television, even copying accents and mannerisms. This was particularly problematic since I was raised on Monty Python, which doesn't always have the most politically correct phrases.

When someone asked me a question, I would have an idea of the kind of answer I wanted to give, but not knowing how to create sentences of my own, I would think back to a response I'd heard on Monty Python, or some other show, that fit the kind of statement and emotion I wanted to express. I would walk up to complete strangers and say the most inappropriate things, and I would do it with a perfect English accent. Can you imagine a four-year-old Canadian boy saying, "Don't give me that, you stupid git!"?

Once while at the grocery store with my mother, I pointed at a chocolate bar I wanted. When my mother said she couldn't get it for me, I called her a "parrot-faced wazzle." She burst out laughing right in the store, because she knew what I was copying.

Why did I do this? It may have been a manifestation of shyness. I knew what I wanted to say, but I didn't want to say it my own way, in case I didn't do it right or was made fun of. I copied what someone else had done because I knew it worked for them. I didn't have to reveal myself or my imperfections by saying something in my own way. It may be similar to the reason for ritualism. I do something the exact same way each time because I know it works, and I'm afraid to try something else.

It's a good thing I didn't have the television series *Lost* as a child, or else every time somebody said something intriguing, I'd reply with, "Hmm... now that's an interesting thing to say—for a heroine addict."

Once, while my mother drove my sister Karen somewhere with me sat in the back seat, out of the blue I started to spout dialogue from the British show *Some Mothers Do 'Ave 'Em*. My mother and sister started laughing immediately, but I was unaware of it so I just went on uninterrupted. My mother had to pull over and park the car because she couldn't stop laughing. I don't know how long it took her to regain her composure once I came to the end of the scene.

I remember once imitating Joan Rivers at the end of one of her shows. Karen saw me and told my mom to watch while I did it again. The same happened when I imitated badly acted commercials. We had a lot of fun.

I once had an argument with my friend over what a movie character had said, so I quoted the entire scene, mannerisms, multiple characters, sound effects, and everything. That shut him up.

Now that I've found my own voice, or one I feel comfortable with, I'm not as good at exact imitation as when I was a kid. At times, that feels like a shame. There are many scenes and commercials I'd like to show the kid inside the younger me so I could watch myself act them out. That would be hilarious!

PACING

As a severe autistic, I often walked in a straight line whether there was a straight path available or not. I had no concept of walking off a cliff or into oncoming traffic. In order to stop me from walking off into the unknown, my mother taught me to walk in a circle around a single object, like a post or box. My habit of walking in circles continued even after I developed an awareness of my surroundings.

This is what started me pacing, which I still do to this day. It's my preferred method of developing and organizing my thoughts. At one point, I remember concluding that I was addicted to pacing, because it was the first thing I did when I got up. Sometimes I would keep going for an hour or two before sitting down to eat or read. It was even my preferred form of entertainment over TV and video games.

These days, pacing is the necessary part of my late evening when I sort through everything that happened that day. Sometimes that can take multiple hours, and it can only be done in isolation.

While working at Karen's store, I spent a lot of time in the back office, just pacing back and forth—which I've discovered isn't as efficient as pacing in a circle, because having to stop and turn around interrupts my thought process. By the time we moved to a new location, the carpet in that office had turned blue from the soles of my sneakers.

PERFORMANCE

Even in my later childhood, I constantly walked into walls and fell down stairs. This was a daily practice, even in public. One day, my teacher called my mother to meet with her while she sat me down for a discussion.

She was convinced that I either needed glasses or was unaware of my surroundings.

When she asked me why I kept walking into walls, my answer was simply, "It makes people laugh."

I was raised on slapstick comedy. I knew what made people laugh and I wanted to bring joy to people, so I walked into walls. My mother and teacher were relieved to hear that, though they suggested I tone it down so I didn't keep scaring people.

One day, I rolled down two flights of stairs in a public building, grunting the whole way. Several people went white-faced as I snowballed down the stairs. My mother, not quite fast enough to grab me before I started rolling, just stood at the top of the stairs shaking her head in resignation. *There he goes again.*

When I hit the floor, I lay still just long enough for the scene to officially end, then jumped to my feet, grinning with satisfaction, and walked out the building with my mother.

Shortly after that, I began a career as an actor.

ORGANIZING

Meticulous organization is a common trait of high-functioning autistics, along with super-active imaginations. I'm past the point of these traits being out of my control. I have the ability to turn them on and off at will.

Organizing is fun. I can't say why. Perhaps it has something to do with precision. The best example I can think of is Pokémon trading cards. I like to arrange them in a certain order, then rearrange them in another order. Sometimes I line them up across the floor in ordered rows and observe them, noting the largest groups and most powerful groups.

Organizing to the extent I do is time-consuming, so I don't do it unless my night is free, or I'm willing to take a break partway through. Even when the job is finished, sometimes I observe my organized display for only a few moments before arranging it another way, not even basking in the joy of completion. The work itself is the most enjoyable part.

Every time I get new cards, I rearrange my display, take stock on my computer, and make piles of duplicates to trade for.

I recently discovered the ability to download music from a CD onto my laptop, and then create personalized playlists. When I discovered this, it was far too late in the night to start, since I had to get up early the next morning. The following day, I scrounged through the house looking for as many music CDs as I could find.

Forming my playlists, I intentionally tried to link the songs together in ways that told a flowing story. I followed Kutless's "In Me" (a song about a guy explaining to his friends why he doesn't hang out at the bar anymore) with Evanescence's "Call Me When You're Sober." I used Chris Daughtry's "Over You" as an immediate follow-up to *The Wedding Singer*'s "Somebody Kill Me Please."

My first mix CD contained mostly songs from Evanescence, Kutless, and Chris Daughtry, with one each from Linkin Park, Savage Garden, and The Smiths.

I can see the forming of playlists becoming a new organizing craze for me, maybe even replacing trading cards. I've already started putting together themed playlists like worship, inspirational, personal, and impressive guitar play.

This Christmas, I asked for a number of music CDs, including Amanda Marshall's self-titled album featuring the song "This Is Love," which has often randomly come on the radio and spoken hope to me when my life was particularly dark. I've decided I want it played at my funeral.

CHANGE-RESISTANT

Change is uncomfortable and scary. I have control over what I know. When things change, my control changes, my sense of security changes. It has taken a lot for me to get to the point where I could honestly say that I trust God. Even now, I struggle.

A change in a plan or routine takes me a moment to adjust to. In the past, I have turned down many opportunities to do something fun and interesting because I couldn't work out in my head how I could get one change to align with the original plan.

I'm more flexible today, though I wouldn't say I'm spontaneous. Even changes in planning require re-planning.

I used to have a pair of jeans with a hole in the crotch… and a bloodstain. It took me a while to get rid of those jeans, and I did so reluctantly. I figured they were a conversation starter.

I do have a particular spot where I like to sit, but I'm physically capable of sitting somewhere else if need be. I don't know why, but I've been met with fear when I've walked into the living room and discovered someone sitting in that particular spot. I don't say anything to them, but I do pause a moment to decide where else to sit. I'm unaware of doing anything hostile toward these people. Is it possible that my face activates an emotion without my knowledge?

INNER THOUGHTS

Most people admit to having inner conversations with themselves, but not the way I do. While most people have mental arguments, or are put down by inner "voices," I was taught long ago where negative thoughts originate, and I learned not to listen. Plus, with God, I know how to get rid of them.

The kinds of conversations I have with myself are just that—conversations. There's some debate as to whether I'm talking with God, my spirit, or just using creativity to play both sides of a discussion. At any one time, it could be a combination of the above. Sometimes I picture a specific person I know, as a preparation for what I intend to say when I see them next. Most of the time talking to myself is a strategy to deal with my thoughts in a constructive manner.

The practice of playing both sides of a discussion comes from a strategy I've employed to allow me to defend both sides of an argument. I'm not a particularly good debater, at least not in the sense of wit. My response time is too slow for live debate. My programming is to process all knowledge, no matter how extensive the process, and come to a sound conclusion only when the research has been completed. It's against my nature to rush to an answer that's only partially conceived.

That's why I hate the prospect of "debate" over "discussion." In a debate, your objective is to choose a side and stick with it, even when your own research proves you wrong. But a discussion is a group effort with lots of people offering different facts, putting them together as one whole study for the purpose of coming to the discovery of a mutual truth.

My thought process is perfectly suited for a discussion. If I don't have an answer, I feel no shame in admitting that, then doing the research until the answer is found.

However, not everyone I meet wants to discuss things; they want to debate. Because there are countless issues I care deeply about in this world, which are under constant attack due to "facts," I feel it necessary to discuss these issues with myself, defending both sides of the argument. This is a scary prospect sometimes, because in all honesty the immediate facts aren't always in my favour—at least not until further research is done.

I have intentionally explored the evidence for other belief systems, realizing that at some point I had to know I had given them a fair chance. Many people believe what they believe only because it's what they grew up with. Then their world falls apart at the first challenge. I had to put my faith to the test so I would know I had a reason to believe what I believe.

At first, I was timid in my questioning. I have often been afraid to acknowledge the questions in my mind, afraid God would be offended and see them as a lack of faith. In fact, the opposite is true—I offend Him by not asking, showing a lack of faith in His ability to answer.

The next challenge for me was understanding the pain people live with, the kind of pain that makes their belief system seem like the only truth. My problem is that I lack empathy and have an over-logical mind; I have been praying for God to mend both. A purely logical mind has its place, I know. I also know that I wouldn't be given a mind like this if not for a purpose. But it's not the right tool for healing broken hearts.

When someone asks me why I believe what I believe, I can give them logical, scientific, historical, and personal reasons, but I don't always discern why they ask, and without knowing I can't determine the manner in which to give the answer. I don't know the kind of answer their hurting soul needs to hear.

While in my early teens, I remember having an argument with my mom, an argument which I either won or believed I'd won because I got the last word. After a few minutes of silence, I admitted, "You know, I've noticed that I sometimes make an argument and then continue to defend it even after I've realized it's wrong."

I think she said something like, "That's common for people." Or perhaps it was more like, "I'm aware of that."

CHAPTER TWO

My Origin Story

MY FAMILY

My parents grew up in Keighly, West Yorkshire, England. He was a farmboy and her family owned a business. She got caught up in the hippy craze of the mid 60s, though she was unable to attend Woodstock and never got into the "enlightenment" lifestyle—or so she tells me. They met at a young farmer's youth group and my father fell in love with her. But her family moved to Canada before he proposed, so he proposed via love letters.

My mother moved back to England for the wedding, but because Canada had become her home, their married life actually began in Toronto. That's where they had their first child—Anna.

But my father's heart was still in England. He hadn't settled to life in Canada, so they moved back to the English farm for half a year before getting their own little house, where they had Karen.

The family entered into a difficult time and my mother moved back to Canada with the girls, this time finding a small house in the town of Ajax, Ontario. It was some time before my father followed them. After reconnecting, they settled into family life in Ajax.

Four weeks into my mother's third pregnancy, there were signs that a miscarriage might occur. She took the time to rest as much as she could and entrusted the child to God, praying it would live. If the child would suffer too much, she trusted God would take it home.

Further into the pregnancy, she had a dream where she gave birth to another girl, and this one had a birthmark in the shape of a rose. She took the dream as a sign that God would bless the pregnancy. My parents were hoping for a boy, to name "Benjamin" (after my great-grandfather), but my mother told my father that if it came out a girl they had to call her Rose. Throughout the pregnancy, I was called "Benjamin Rose," because they had no idea which I would be.

When my mother went for an examination, the doctor told her she had a placenta previa, meaning that the placenta was attached to the bottom of the uterus instead of near the top, which also meant there was a good chance my weight would push the placenta out prematurely and I would not survive. For my sake, my mother went on bedrest for a few weeks until all signs were normal. After that, my mother was able to return to her part-time job at the YMCA. For the rest of the pregnancy, however, she was deemed "high risk."

At seven months, I had gotten so big that my mother had to go back on bedrest to prevent gravity from taking over. After a second examination, she discovered that the placenta had moved over a little.

My due date came... and went. Apparently I was quite comfortable staying where I was. The specialist decided to induce my mother the following Monday.

My mother went into labour while watching *Flipper*. Even though I was on my way out, I really didn't want to come, so my mother was induced again to keep things moving. She hadn't dilated enough for a natural birth and a last-minute examination revealed that there was soft tissue where my head was supposed to be in the birth canal. The specialist decided to perform a C-section.

When I came out, the umbilical cord was wrapped around my neck, preventing me from getting the necessary oxygen. The doctor was able to help me recover, though—and I was huge! Ten pounds, five ounces. The nurses named me "Big Ben." Even with four nephews and a niece, I still proudly hold the title of "Frickin' Hugest Baby" in my family.

And so I was born on December 15, 1983.

CHILDHOOD

My earliest memories consist of four things.

1. Playing with a toy called "Barrel of Monkeys." I actually remember wondering whether this was the product everyone referred to when they said, "More fun than a barrel of monkeys."

2. Vomiting. The smell is etched into my memory, which is why to this day I cannot eat a certain type of Hamburger Helper, nor certain types of cheese.

3. Playing with Batman and Robin figurines that came with detachable capes. The capes had hard collars that snap off at the back of the neck. I used to take those off and pretend they were manta rays attacking capeless Batman and Robin. I don't remember who won, but probably the manta ray/capes, since as a child I always favoured creatures over people.

4. My warmest memory is sitting inside the living room toy chest watching *Thunder Cats*. I remember the weird mummy guy and wondering why he was only taped-up half the time. I remember that the toy I wanted most was the furry white ape guy.

As a child, my autism was severe. I couldn't sit still, I couldn't listen, and I couldn't communicate. I had no sense of danger, no sense of other people, and no sense of my environment. My sisters, however, will attest that I was very cute.

In my toddler years, I was obsessed with ponytails. My first steps were to grab a girl's ponytail.

The first dream I can remember took place after I fell asleep in the basement. I dreamt of cartoonish characters, kind of like man-sized Muppets. It was one of those dreams that felt familiar, but I've since learned that dreams can provide false memories. I don't know if I had met those characters in my dreams before, but they felt familiar.

Being in this dream was like being in an episode of a kid's TV show. The dream I remember was the Halloween special and everyone was actually someone else. Everybody looked normal until they unzipped their costumes and revealed themselves to be somebody else. The plump yellow guy was actually the red guy, the one human was actually the

21

yellow guy, and the red guy was actually the green giant with pigtails. I don't remember if I was disguised or not.

BARRIERS

In my years of severe autism, I walked into things on a regular basis. As I gradually developed an awareness of my surroundings, I got to the point where I knew enough to stop when I walked up to a closed door. But that was it. Once I stopped in front of a shut door, I didn't know what else to do. I knew there was a way people got these things to move, but I didn't understand that power or how to get it.

I had the same reaction to walls. I knew they were an obstruction, but I wasn't sure how to get past them. I also wondered why people didn't move these things the way they moved doors. It took a while before I realized that doors and walls were different things.

PLAYING WITH LIGHT

During the day, I would lie in bed or on the couch and make the sunlight do weird things by squinting my eyes or tilting my head different ways. I found that if the light was on me and I squinted my eyes just enough, the light would stretch into a thin beam shooting up and down from its source. Squint a bit more and I could see microscopic life forms slide slowly down the surface of my vision.

I would take the cardboard back of toy blister packs, grab a push-pin, and poke holes in the eyes of every character on the back of the board. Then I'd hold it up against the sun and see the light shine through the tiny holes. Everyone's eyes would glow.

When I saw two objects, one very close to my face and the other some distance behind it, I found that focusing on one object made the other split into two. I made a habit of using this knowledge to duplicate objects and tilt my head to make them dance around each other.

Even a stain on the windshield became something to play with. By focusing on the road lines, I could make a single dead bug or crack become two and then try to keep the lines in between the two without touching. Not while driving, of course.

THE COLOURS

At night, in the darkness, the world would be alive with colours. Not a plethora of colours but a mixture of reds and yellows, pinks and oranges. They were extremely erratic and annoying, constantly moving like a buzzing hive of colours, never settling down.

It was the same when I closed my eyes. Actually, it was worse. With my eyes closed, the colours came in waves, this time including greens, blues, and purples. Like shockwaves emanating from the centre of my vision, with something like colourful static all around. I found that with my eyes closed I could focus on the dead centre of my vision and find depth in what I saw, piercing into spacious worlds of darkness and colour.

I eventually realized that these buzzing colours weren't exclusive to the darkness. Even in brightest daylight, if I looked at a surface that was all one colour, the buzzing was there as well. The buzzing is all around, everywhere, all the time. It's simply less noticeable when I'm already looking at a complexity of colours in the world around me. Even now, if I stare at anything, or close my eyes, the buzzing is there, but I no longer notice it unless I focus.

Normally the buzzing was too erratic to do anything with, but some nights they came together and took shape. One night, a giant face or skull appeared above my bed and descended upon me with its mouth wide open to swallow me. Even back then, I fought against such things. I kicked up my feet as it came down. I don't know if it drew back or went right through me, but another one appeared to try to swallow me again.

At the time, I didn't know how to dispel these kinds of attacks. Since the faces wouldn't stop, I got out of bed and went to sleep on the living room couch. I kept my eye on the hall to see if anything was following me; the usual buzz of colours was in the living room as well. Eventually, I perceived a slow-motion flood of intense colours pouring out from the hall to scare me on the couch. I don't remember what I did after that; whether it was that night or later on, I eventually realized that the thick clusters of colours couldn't harm me. I learned either to live with them or ignore them.

THE CHRISTIAN HOUSEHOLD

My entire family is Christian. The basis of the faith made sense to me, but my introduction to religion was through a very conservative church. This was an uncomfortable fit for someone who was genuinely unaware of rules.

School was worse, with having to stay there practically the whole day. Very few teachers understood what my needs were, or why I was this way. I repeatedly disturbed the classroom and didn't even know it.

I was raised mainly by my mother, with my two sisters stepping in when she was busy. My father worked full days, and even when he was home he wasn't a social person and never connected with me emotionally. I do recall him trying now and then to connect with me over coffee and juice, or with a game of catch, but I didn't know who he was. I tended to respond to him as a stranger who had my mother's permission to be with me for a few hours.

In my later years I knew who he was, and I developed some emotional need I didn't understand. But we never made a strong father-son connection.

It's come out in recent conversations with him, and with the rest of the family, that my father likely also has a condition lying somewhere on the autism spectrum. His condition has never been as serious as mine, and it hasn't interfered with his ability to work, but it has made socializing a challenge for him. I've also recently come to realize how often autistic traits are passed down to one's children, though the severity can be different from one generation to the next.

I don't remember much of my life before age four, but my mother and sister report that it was in that year that I let Jesus into my life. As a result, I don't have a grand conversion story as some people have when they give their lives to Christ later in life. I didn't have the experience of my whole outlook changing within days or months. Instead my life has been a gradual, progressive discovery of what life as a Christian means.

While some people get the immediate sense of becoming a guiding light for others, I was twelve before I felt that sense of purpose. While some people realize right away why they no longer need to be perfectionists, it took me until my twenty-second year to even realize that

I *was* a perfectionist; immediately I realized I didn't need to be. While some people report immediate feelings of excitement, unburdening, and acceptance, I still struggle with those feelings to this day. While still others report immediate feelings of closeness with God, and everything suddenly making sense, I have to confess that I've had those feelings all my life. In spite of the good, the bad, and the ugly, life to me has never made sense without God in the equation.

My mother once gave me a picture book about the Creation, which contained the story of Adam and Eve and the serpent. One page had an illustration of Satan, which was just a bald head with dark eyes and a smile. I didn't understand how a smile could be evil, but since this was my first image of what evil supposedly looked like, I developed an intolerance of bald people who smiled too much. I later grew out of that... although the Emperor from *Star Wars* fortified that intolerance for many years.

The first theological question I had was, "If God forgives us, why doesn't He forgive Satan?" It was a genuine question, but I think I took it to a cynical level, as happened in those years. My mother was delighted to hear that question, and encouraged me to ask the pastor directly next Sunday.

My mother led me through the church, up to the pastor, and prompted me to ask my question. I did. But in all honesty, I don't recall a word that was spoken. This was the first time I ever saw the pastor up close, you see, and he was an old man. Words came out of him, but I was so struck by the amount of visual information on his face that I was overstimulated.

My mother testifies that even as a severe autistic I was very open to God's presence in my life. At times when she couldn't help me, she could somehow get through to me the message, "I can't help you, but ask God for help." I would ask, and whatever problem I was having, He would help me with it, and I would be okay.

CHAPTER THREE
The Learning Process

SCHOOL

We'll call the public school I went to "South Park," though obviously that's not its real name.

In preschool, my favourite thing to do was play with the ponytail of whichever girl was sitting in front of me. This got me into trouble and the teacher often had to sit me in a corner away from class. (Discipline never worked on me because I didn't know why I was being punished). So I left the room to play in the sandbox outside, which infuriated the teacher.

She apparently didn't see anything different about me and insisted that I was simply more disobedient than the other kids. My mother and her got into a lot of arguments about how to communicate with me.

"He doesn't pay attention when I say 'Class'!"

"That's because his name isn't 'Class'!"

Looking back at it, my preschool teacher was a nasty piece of work. That's one of the few memories of eye contact that I have from that time, one of the first visions of pure rage. I got the impression that she had issues. In fact, later in life I found out that she had a nervous breakdown; it happened after I left for grade school, though, so it wasn't *all* me.

Grade One was awkward. It wasn't in my nature to sit still or hang out with other kids or have an interest in math. My oversensitive hearing also made it hard to stay in class, with all the running and screaming of other kids. I kept getting ear infections, which of course made the sensitivity worse. Even when I sat at my desk, I couldn't focus on a lesson because of all the distractions.

To make matters worse, there were actually two classes in one room at the same time. I liked the other class better, so I kept walking across the room to sit with the other kids.

My teachers' general complaints about me included moping, crying, screaming, aggressive behaviour, hitting, and failure to follow instructions. All of which are appropriate complaints. They also had concerns about my non-social tendencies, my ability to hold the pencil right, and my tendency to be too focused on specific subjects. At times, I wouldn't want to go outside for recess because I preferred in-class activities to the swings. I threw a tantrum whenever activity time ended too quickly—this may have been the beginning of my hatred for time limits, and my anxiety at beginning tasks that I know will take time.

From time to time, I took tests designed to assess my development. When asked, "Where's your shoe?" I answered, "On my sock." This was regarded as an inappropriate answer.

Reading didn't go over well, because in those days they were teaching kids to read words by memory, which my brain couldn't wrap itself around. My mother taught me phonics during summer vacation and I learned that way, but when I got back to school they told me I couldn't do it that way and they forced me back into their method of teaching. And so I forgot how to read.

Though I was lacking in several categories, I excelled at story writing and illustrations. This was one of the few areas where I actually got praise from teachers.

One time, we were asked to draw a picture, but before I finished the teachers announced that time was up and we were to move on to the next subject. I couldn't do that. I hadn't finished. One by one, kids were sent over to get me to stop and I told them to leave and let me finish. The last kid actually pushed my hand while I was drawing and made me ruin my work. Seeing my work destroyed, I had a fit of rage and scribbled aggressively on the kid's back. Poor guy. I don't remember how sharp the pencil was, but there were no apparent injuries.

I remember the first time I drew a creature in class. It was a creature of my own invention and had its own lifestyle. I immediately thought, "I'm as good as God if I can create things!" In my mind, imagining something was the same as God physically creating it. That first creature was very simplistic—it was blue and lizard-like—but I was very proud.

Shortly afterward, I invented a predatorial hedgehog that was green so it looked like grass and could sneak up on other creatures. I was so proud of myself that I continued to invent creatures with the ability to hide by looking like the things around them. Bet God never thought of that!

I was in music class once. Only once. It was a nightmare, being surrounded by kids with the loudest possible instruments making what I could only interpret as a lot of noise. I insisted on being far away, and again teachers would talk to me or send kids to try talking me into participating. I would tell them I couldn't. I think someone told me, "Just do it!" After a few minutes of balancing my need to be away with my need to rid myself of guilt, I walked into the band, picked up the first instrument I found, and started participating in the noise. I was immediately taken off-stage and told to stay far away.

I kept getting lost at school. It was very big, and when there weren't other kids to follow back to class, I got lost. I remember one time being asked by a teacher to deliver something to the principal. I don't remember how, but I made it to his office and gave him the letter. Afterward, I stood around with a perplexed look on my face. Somehow I ended up having lunch with the guy and some of his associates. We had pizza. I don't even remember when my parents picked me up, but I think they came to the restaurant to get me.

In my later years, I've been trying hard to remember the details of that day, wondering if I was in trouble for something. Did the principal just want to see me for some reason? Was there, in fact, something terrible that happened that day? The main thing I recall is the feeling I had about this man, that he had no idea what was up with me, but he apparently liked me and wasn't too proud to have this kid he'd just met sitting with him and his associates.

Thinking on it now, it's entirely possible that I was given instructions on how to get to this man's office, but not instructions on how to get back to class. When he asked me the name of my teacher, I didn't know, so the guy probably had no choice but to take me with him to this business meeting while the school secretary asked around for a teacher who had Benjamin Collier in their class.

There was one place, though, which I definitely knew how to get to—home.

The whole school-recess-school thing never made sense to me. One day around lunchtime, my mom saw me walk into the house and begin playing on the floor. She called the school to ask if I had been sent home. The school was dumbfounded. During recess, I had walked home from school *on my own*. They demanded that she drive me back to school, but she said no. "For the sake of two hours? Just so you can lose him again? Get your act together."

One progress report from the academic resource teacher went like this:

> Ben finds it difficult to express his feelings. He constructed a puppet bearing a happy face on one side and a sad face on the other. Using this puppet he was then able to identify his feelings in given situations. Ben has demonstrated some very creative work.

The majority of the public school board, and the church, told my mother that the best thing to do was put me on Ritalin, believing that my trouble paying attention in class and church was simply due to an overdose of energy. She refused. My mother was convinced that God had allowed me to be this way for a reason. Changing me would be to take away God's plan for who I was meant to be. As it was put in the movie *Super Star*, "If God gave [him] excess energy, then by God, nobody's taking it from [him]."

Everyone believed me to be a hopeless case, that nothing could come of me. Apparently the only thing to do was stop me from causing any more problems. My mother's response went like this: "Wait and see what God will do with this child."

CORRECTIONAL SCHOOL

After I repeated Grade One and still couldn't move forward, it was clear that something had to change. The school board was convinced that what I needed was a behavioural correction school, so they sent me to Dunder Mifflin (again, not real name). This meant leaving behind all my friends at South Park and the girl who I considered to be my girlfriend.

The teachers in my new class were all women, and similar in personality to my preschool teacher, as I would soon discover. Only they were far more experienced.

Dunder Mifflin had a merit system. You would get smiley faces for being good and frowny faces for being bad. I didn't understand what they considered "good" as opposed to "bad," nor was it ever properly explained to me—all I knew was that as I sat at my desk trying to behave the teachers would walk by my desk and put a frowny face on my paper without telling me why. At least I knew that it took three frownies a day to be bad, so the first two I got didn't concern me, just confused me. But when the third one appeared, I couldn't believe it. I was genuinely shocked to discover that I was a bad kid—I would never have thought so otherwise.

One time, while walking down the hall alone, probably on an errand for a teacher, a bigger kid walked up to me and stood in my way. When I tried to get around him, he moved in front of me again. I growled, and then he let me pass without further trouble. The possibility of being beaten up had never even occurred to me.

Another time as I was walking down the hall on my own, a kid spotted me and said, "Ben Collier? *You* don't belong here." He must have known me from South Park, but I couldn't remember faces very well. I just looked at him with resignation and said, "Yes, I do."

Apparently there was some great concern over me not knowing how to tie shoelaces. This problem was easily solved when my mother bought me a pair of Velcro shoes, but the teachers were insistent that learning to tie shoelaces was an essential part of my education. Every morning I would miss the beginning of class because one of the teachers would keep me outside, take off my Velcro shoes, and put a laced pair on me in a vain attempt to show me how it's done. Even the way I tied my shoes was wrong.

It was while at this school, around the building and on the bus there and back, that I discovered things like mean-spirited sarcasm, the "FU" handsign, and certain sexual acts.

After a while, I decided one day to try being bad on purpose, just to see what it felt like. At the time, this consisted only of insulting people. My punishment was to spend time in detention, which was a boring waste of time. I decided I didn't like being bad. The problem was that even after making the decision to be good, I found that I couldn't stop being bad—I was still getting frowny faces for unknown reasons. I couldn't help it.

Everyday when I got home I would shut myself in my room for hours and not talk to anyone. It took me that long to unwind from a day of school.

I was seven and still hadn't officially been diagnosed with autism, but my mother strongly suspected that this was what I had. She believed that having a diagnosis would help everyone understand what I needed in terms of education.

She started taking me to Sick Children's Hospital, where we connected with a specialist named Mary MacDonald. We had to rename her "Mary Mac" because every time I heard her name I thought I was getting McDonald's.

While seeing her, my mother explained my learning process like this: "He doesn't learn things the same as other children because he seems to need something he already knows to build a new idea on. It's like he's standing at the side of a fast flowing river. The water is information he's trying to collect. The other side is the new idea he's trying to learn. Others would cross over at the bridge, but he can't find a bridge to cross over safely. All he has is stepping stones and it's difficult for him to keep his footing while navigating the fast river. Sometimes he just has to turn back and he gets frustrated and angry at himself for not being able to get across. Then sometimes he makes it and he's so pleased! Each stepping stone has to be something he already knows, and then he can step onto it. Then he has to find another stone that he already knows, and so on, until he reaches the other side. Most people don't have to work that hard at every single new thing they learn."

From this description, Mary MacDonald concluded that I had not autism, but something called Asperger's Syndrome, what some would call "high-functioning autism."

My mother was relieved to finally have an answer. But what to do about my education?

One day while I was completing an extra assignment for disciplinary purposes, one of the teachers came up to me. "Ben, how old are you?" When I told her my age, she said, "Well, that looks like three-year-old writing."

By that time, I was thoroughly convinced that I hated these women.

I myself don't have memory of this, but my mother reports that up until then I only drew in black and white. This was the first year I ever drew using colour, and its first occurrence was in a drawing of all the kids and teachers shooting each other between buildings—heads flying and blood spurting everywhere. Bright red.

Going through some of my old schoolwork recently, I found the picture she was referring to, and looking at the picture now it is unclear exactly how upset I was at the time I drew it. All the faces, even the decapitated ones, are smiling. I can see my humour in it. I did this drawing three times, and in two of them I'm in the air with a parachute or balloon. In one of the drawings my head was shot off, and in another I'd been shot in the stomach. It occurs to me, however, that I'm not holding any kind of weapon in any of them.

As my mom picked me up from school one day (I was banned from the bus for bad behaviour), she asked me if I wanted to stay at Dunder Mifflin or if I would rather she taught me at home.

It didn't take me long to answer.

HOME-SCHOOLING

My mother had experience teaching grade school, so she was qualified to be my private teacher for the time being—as long as she stuck to the available curriculum.

Math and English were pretty straightforward, but Science had a number of possible avenues. Every time we picked up a new Science book, my mom would let me choose the subjects. Can you imagine how my heart rose when I discovered I could study dinosaurs for school? Dinosaurs were my subject of choice for some considerable time, broken only occasionally by an interest in space.

On the cover of my Grade Two space book was a picture of a crescent moon with an astronaut-bear standing on it. As far as astrophysics goes, this taught me that the moon was hook-shaped, just big enough for one bear to fit inside, and if you stood on it, gravity would pull you toward the bottom of it.

For reading time, I often selected Choose-Your-Own-Adventure books. My interest in how particular decisions would lead to particular events kept me reading beyond the required time. I would look up the results of every possible choice.

Since my mom had me for the whole day, she started off every morning with prayer and Bible reading. I remember this being awkward, and it may have been the start of me feeling uncomfortable praying out loud in a group. There was a rule that I had to think of something to thank God for every time I prayed to Him, but I didn't always feel thankful. (Of course, considering where I'd come from, I had a lot to be thankful for, but as a kid you live in the moment). It felt wrong to say to God something I was being told to feel instead of what I actually felt, so I didn't like talking to God out loud while other people listened, judging my reasons for saying this or that.

I tended to feel stupid whenever I came across a question I didn't have an answer to. At the time, it was beyond me to reason, "I only don't know this because nobody's told me about it yet." When I finally realized that knowledge could be gained by asking someone, reading about it, or watching a documentary, I became a sponge.

This is a lesson I've had to relearn several times in life. When someone uses a word or phrase I'm unfamiliar with, it has become natural for me to ask them about it, admitting, "I've never heard that before" or "I've heard that here and there, but I haven't figured out what it means."

Just last night, I texted my friend to ask what T&A is. When he told me, I said, "Oh, I knew that! I thought it was something more elaborate."

Apparently my mom got me to read through the television. Whenever I asked what was on, she'd tell me she was too busy to read the TV Guide—so I did.

I can act, draw, and write. I have done all three, but I don't know how they can be put to use in one project, so right now I'm focusing on writing. Although I took up drawing, I've only attempted to take an art class twice. I got through the first class with no problems. What put me off in the second was being told to draw the shapes of the things I wanted to draw. Drawing shapes just got in the way for me. I saw it as a waste.

"BOGOSITY"

Many adults in authority positions have had problems with me. The second time I took art class, I drew a picture and added a little extra thing to make my friends laugh. It turned out that what I added to the picture was inappropriate, which I didn't know until the teacher told me. But instead of simply telling me, he swiped the picture from me and gave me a lecture on inappropriate behaviour in front of the class. After which I said, "You could have just asked me to erase it."

He was very obviously embarrassed, and I didn't know why. I was only giving him advice on how to improve his teaching. It was only fair, since he had informed me of what kind of drawings were inappropriate, which I genuinely hadn't known before and would then keep in mind.

My ability to see logic and failures of logic has always made certain adults uncomfortable, as well as my ability to see past the facades that people construct to make themselves appear faultless—what I've heard Jack Black refer to as "bogosity." Some teachers just didn't know how to deal with me.

In my observation of social interaction, I have discovered two types of power: ego and ignorance.

Ego power is based on aggressive, self-promoting behaviour. It relies on everyone acknowledging it, and no one stronger challenging it. Someone with ego power needs to express their power in order to feel it. They need to butt heads, they need to speak loud, they need to impose. There are places where this kind of power is useful, particularly when bringing calm to a chaotic group of people, or when a good man with ego power challenges a man abusing his power.

Ignorance power is anti-ego, being automatically unaware of anyone's ego power, or at least not perceiving it as a threat. Ignorance is dependent on not getting caught up in the temptation to challenge ego. People with ignorance power don't need to give their power expression; they exude power simply by their presence and a kind of inner calm, which comes in handy when a person with nothing but ego is trying to get a rise out of you.

Each power has its strengths and weaknesses. Someone with ego power loses their power when someone completely ignores them, but gains even more power if they manage to get a rise out of everyone. Likewise, people with ignorance power can look even more powerful than all the egotistical loudmouths around them, but only as long as they manage to remain undisturbed. If they fail to ignore, they lose their ignorance power and the egos gain even more.

I don't think it's a rule that a person has either one power or the other. I think it's possible for one person to succeed at both. But our personalities and preferences cause us to lean toward one or the other, or fluctuate between the two depending on the situation.

As someone with ignorance power, I have made a lot of egotistical people look stupid. When I try to take over a room, I fail miserably, and some egotistical people have been very distraught simply by having me in the room. I've been in a classroom with a teacher who's been afraid of me simply because I was there. I make no move to take power from these people, but they react to my presence as if I'm going to.

I remember watching cartoons or puppet shows on TV, and every time a real adult would come onscreen I'd feel a sense of violation. Cartoons are innocent, puppets are innocent, but adults aren't. I always felt like a world of complete innocence was being violated by masked evil when a real adult walked on, creating an environment of pretension.

I was never abused as a child, as far as I remember. I think the reason for this line of thought was just that adults always feigned innocence around me, refusing to admit imperfection. My own careful research of adult life, however, which I carried out when they thought I wasn't looking, revealed the true nature of every adult heart. This was one reason I never wanted to grow up. I knew that no matter how hard I tried to remain innocent, I would become like them. I would commit evil.

Of course I did grow up, reluctantly. But as I did, I made a promise to myself to never forget what I learned as a child, to never give in to hypocrisy. If I'm going to be imperfect, I shouldn't act as though I'm perfect. I would never swear or make coarse jokes in front of children, but neither would I act as though I never swear at all.

When talking with my young nephews, I have actual conversations with them. I don't speak in child or baby tongue. I speak at my level. I think that's one reason why kids like me so much; I treat them like equals. I don't pretend to be innocent when I'm around them because I remember what it felt like to have adults do that to me. It made me feel like I couldn't trust them. A person who openly admits imperfection is a person you can trust.

I realized recently that this continuing desire to not betray childhood is a matter of patriotism. Childhood is where I started out; therefore, it's my native land. Time forced me into a different land before I was ready to leave, but I still try to speak the native tongue (honesty) when I'm around children. I'm attempting to be a dual citizen.

During his lecture, that art teacher told me, "Feel free to draw this kind of filth at home, but not in my class." Unfortunately, I took his advice. That night, I drew a picture so disturbing that when I stumbled upon it years later I couldn't believe an eight-year-old had drawn it. I immediately tore it up.

But I remember right after drawing it, looking at my work and thinking, "This isn't me. I don't like this. I don't enjoy it. I'm not a bad kid after all."

One of the prime captions of my childhood has been grown-ups telling me I'm an inherently bad child, and making me believe it. By staring my own potential for evil in the face and recognizing that I didn't like it, I finally realized I wasn't a bad child; I just didn't fit another person's idea of "good."

Another thing that created a rift between me and adults was my awareness that they all refused to admit they didn't fit their own idea of "good," either. I'm pretty sure my awareness of adult imperfection was just a behavioural observation, noting that who they were when they talked to me was different than who they were when they talked to other adults. I don't have the ability to see into other people's souls—no more than anyone else, anyway. I just analyze. Although I've been told that my stare makes people feel like I'm looking into their soul, I'm actually not. I just have really cool eyes.

Inconsistency is one of the scariest things for a child. If you're shouting and swearing to someone on the phone, then hang up and say to your child, "What's the matter, sweetie? My little baby pumkin schnookums?" This is a very scary moment for a child, because they no longer know who you are.

I don't like it when someone tells me a dirty joke in front of kids. Even if the kid doesn't understand the joke, they do understand that they're being ignored. They understand when adults intentionally talk in a language the child can't interpret and then pretend they didn't say anything at all.

I work hard to establish a level of honesty with the kids I know. I don't like being put in a position where that honesty is compromised.

CHAPTER FOUR

My "Big Kid" Years

We soon moved to another house in Ajax. This time, I managed to make friends on only my second day there. While walking up and down the block on my own, I found a group of younger kids who welcomed me to join them. All the kids I hung out with were two to three years younger than me; they accepted me into their group even though I was a little odd.

Although I became known as "The Christian" in this circle, it was considered a term of endearment and respect. Whatever religions these kids were being raised in, they seemed to acknowledge a greater awareness of God in me than what they were seeing elsewhere. Unfortunately, I didn't know anything about evangelism at the time, so I was unaware of what planting seeds was all about. Maybe they preferred that I was as open as I was without that sense of obligation.

If I had a rebellious stage, then it was very short and very mild. For a couple of months, swearing became part of my regular speech. The horror. But it wasn't long before a revelation came to me that I needed to set a better example. I was the Christian on the block, so I represented Christianity to all the other kids. That's when the rebellious stage ended, if you could call it that.

Matthew, the much respected boss of the group, wanted whatever it was I had, and I attempted to give it to him. "Simply pray to Jesus and let Him into your heart," I said. That was all I understood as a kid; that's probably all any kid can understand about it. I led him through that, but I know he doubted his salvation afterward and I didn't know what else to say. He came to me once and said, "I'm supposed to be Christian now, but I still swear," to which I simply replied, "My dad's Christian and he swears all the time."

Ironically, I quickly developed a reputation among parents as being a "bad influence." This was likely due in part to one couple who perceived my personality to be evil. I know I had similar feelings about them, and questioned them on keeping their kids away from me since we were, at the time, good friends.

At least one of the other kids (at the age of seven) had already seen a porn film (something I would not witness for at least another decade). This kid described the scene to other seven-year-olds in detail. I cared little about this at the time but found it odd that I was the one perceived as being a bad example.

There was one other kid on the street who was my age and came from a correctional school. One day he was bent on teasing and shoving me until I responded, but somehow I responded in the wrong direction and accidentally hurt a little girl. My very first reaction was shock, and worry for the girl, who was clearly hurt. I tried to figure out how the previous chain of events had led to that. Again, nobody understood what was going on with me, and before I could apologize or explain anything the accusations started to fly, much of them coming from the boy who had been pushing me.

Then the girl's mother came out into the street and proceeded to call me a bad person without first going to my parents. Then something new happened. I recognized this to be the same type of woman as those I'd met at Dunder Mifflin. Instead of trying again to clarify what had happened, which I clearly wasn't going to get the chance to do, I stood up to her in front of all my accusers and told her she couldn't judge me.

I don't recall much of the conversation, as even then I was still completely bewildered, but I know she left unsatisfied and said over her shoulder, the way that kind of person does, "He obviously doesn't know how to make friends."

As I was outside in the following days playing with *the friends I had made*, that boy would ride by on his bike and say to me, "Treat people the way you want to be treated." Then he'd do a wheelie and leave. Eventually I asked him if he wanted to be pushed and kicked and teased, and then repeated his quote to him.

He said, "Yeah, wull…"

I didn't hear the rest. I was already walking away.

I later apologized to the girl for hurting her. Of course, it had been my intention to apologize as soon as it happened, but everybody quickly made it into me vs. them and I could do nothing. I later realized this wall they had set up was stupid and was keeping me from doing the right thing. I didn't explain that it was an accident, because to have observed it from afar I wouldn't have believed myself. She forgave me, but I doubt her mother ever did.

That same girl was later in an armcast for something that same boy had done while playing with her. I heard no commotion over that.

I think that was the first time I really understood that there exists in this world a certain type of woman, and that type should always be avoided. That type and me would never get along. My life after that has proven this realization correct. I run into these women everywhere. Church is no exception. Friendship is very difficult to establish with these kinds of women because all they care for is vengeance for any perceived wrong.

This was also the beginning of my realization that I could stand up to them. Despite their power, they lack logic, and as long as logic is on my side, I will always know how illogical these women are. I will know that the things they say, no matter how hurtful, are the wild ravings of illogical creatures. Knowing this has helped me walk away from many nasty women without compromising myself.

Around that time, I invented a game called "Be Whoever You Want to Be." While playing with my friends, instead of limiting our character selection to the Ninja Turtles or Power Rangers, we could take our pick from any movie or show, the only exception being that those you played with had to understand your character and his or her parameters.

In later years, I used this as an excuse to test my creativity and invent new characters to play as. As long as I could sufficiently explain the kind of character I was playing, I was permitted to use him; the other kids knew the difference between real creativity and playing god. One of my friends once pretended to spray something at me, and because I knew my character had large eyes I pretended that the spray had temporarily blinded me; this was received as "cool," and people became very interested in this character of mine.

MEGAN

The first girl I considered a "girlfriend" was Megan. I didn't know much about relationships at the age of six, but I remember being completely paralyzed at the first sight of her, and understanding that such a reaction could only be love. For a time, we went to South Park together. I once put together an odd drawing and attached a candy cane to it; I gave it to her, the first indication that I liked her. I don't remember much of what we did together except that we sat together a lot.

Things got complicated once I started seeing how badly my sisters' boyfriends treated them. I didn't know what relationships were supposed to be like, so I drew from the only examples I had, which didn't go over well.

When I started at Dunder Mifflin, I couldn't see her as much. The distance between us continued to grow, even on the few occasions we did see each other.

Although when I moved to this new house, I was geographically closer to Megan, we didn't see each other very often. The little time we spent together made us feel too different in terms of interests. I still didn't know what a relationship was supposed to be like and I didn't know what was expected of me. By then, I'd begun feeling pressure to do things right, becoming defensive when I felt I was missing the mark.

The thing I blamed myself most for was my pride. I had it in mind that a girlfriend could not be older than a boyfriend, so every time we met I asked how old she was. It didn't occur to me that I could ask her age and then ask her birthday and that would be that. I think she was offended that I repeated the same question every time.

At the age of ten, I made her a Valentine's Day card and delivered it to her in person. By then I had seen so little of her and we were both growing and changing so fast that I didn't know what to say when I saw her. I had become afraid of what love meant. I believe I came across as cold and careless, but that was my defence for feeling incompetent. That was the last I saw of her.

I kick myself every time I think about it. She was so beautiful when I first met her; even to a six-year-old she stirred up romantic emotion. I can only imagine how beautiful she must be today. I was captivated by her every time we met.

SHANKS

My best friend goes by the name Shanks. I was probably nine by the time I first got to know him, and he would have been six. The age difference didn't bother me because I could only socialize with people either younger than me or older—never peers.

Shanks and I were not exactly alike, but were both equally separate from the rest of the world, and both much further along than others in terms of intellect. As we grew into our twenties, we gradually became what most people would consider peers, but in our eyes we always had been.

By his own confession, his initial reason for wanting to hang out with me was that I was amusing. One day, as all the kids were playing, I ran down the street shouting, "Look! No bike!"

Nobody else got it, but Shanks did. We later found that we shared a lot of random humour most people just didn't get.

Out of all the friends I made on that street, Shanks was the only one I managed to maintain contact with after my next move. Shanks and I have been friends now for eighteen years, almost two-thirds of my life.

Shanks was one of those kids who wanted whatever it was I had with God. He finally made the jump to Christianity when we were in our teens. He has thanked me numerous times for leading him to Christ.

How did I do it? I have no idea. I can tell you that it wasn't through pressure or debating; he's a much better debater than I am. All I can see is that I set the example simply through being me, living openly and honestly. He made the decision himself to become Christian.

I don't think winning a debate has ever led anyone to Christ. You shouldn't have to argue with someone about the difference Christ has made in your life. If you have the joy of salvation, nobody can argue with that; they can only sit back and wonder.

When Shanks found out I was autistic, it came as a total shock to him.

"I had no idea you were autistic!" he said.

"I specifically remember telling you before."

"I thought you were kidding!"

"Didn't you ever question why I have a drawer full of magazine cutouts? Cuz if I saw that in someone else's house, I'd be concerned."

Since then, he's held me up as a prime example to other people of how, through God, one can break free of their supposed limitations.

In my big kid and early teen years, I was bombarded with nasty thoughts that I found difficult to get rid of. Knowing where these thoughts came from, I mentally told them to go away. I was an adult before I realized that such commands had to be spoken aloud and in the name of Jesus. At the time, I had an imaginary robot come in and shoot the nasty thoughts to pieces. That usually helped; imagining minigun fire was a very distracting thought.

THE COUNTRY

I was fourteen when we decided to move again. My two sisters were heading out to an apartment of their own, so we didn't need as big of a house. I think we were starting to get sick of some of the neighbours.

We found a bungalow out in the country that rather reminded my father of growing up on the farm. The backyard was a forest, with a river running through it, and just behind the house was a two-car garage with a shed attachment. But I think what we all fell in love with most was the isolation.

There was one addition to the house that at the time was being used as a rec room. When we moved in, my parents converted it into a new master bedroom—which meant I got the original master bedroom for myself.

One problem was that, upon arrival, we could find no churches around that adhered to the teachings we had been brought up with. It was a year or two before we attended church again.

Around this time, my home-schooling took a turn. My mother was only qualified to teach grade school. To finish my education at the high school level I would have to either go back to public school or take correspondence education. Again, my mother gave me a choice, asking if I felt I needed to be around kids my age. I said no. I genuinely didn't like the idea, nor did I expect to be able to concentrate in a full classroom. The results of not being around peers wouldn't bother me until years later.

Taking a slightly more public form of education also meant that I now had to endure exams—and they were to be timed. Time limits have always been an issue for me, so my mom gave me yet another choice—I could complete the course as is or ask for a time addition handicap. I decided to do it by the set standard. I again needed to know that I could function as a part of the world instead of asking for slack all the time. One benefit of these particular courses was that the exam results didn't have as much of a bearing on the overall results as they do in public schools. This relieved a lot of the tension, but I still tended to suck at finals.

THE YOUTH GROUP

My eldest sister Anna started attending Whitby Baptist Church, which is where she met Josh Sklar, the youth pastor. They were married within a year. Anna became a youth helper and my mom and I started attending the Sunday morning services. I was also convinced to join the youth group.

Even by age fifteen, my social skills hadn't improved. I didn't know how to smile or be "part of the group." I attended and enjoyed the lessons, but afterward when everyone ran to the gym for a game I would look for an adult to assist in whatever capacity was needed. If no help was needed, I'd find a place of my own to sit or pace.

I felt no camaraderie with the guys, only with Josh, who saw the lack of initiation in my life and tried to take me under his wing. Many of his heartfelt attempts fell on deaf ears, though. I was too unfamiliar with what he was doing to understand the purpose, and it didn't help that we were two completely different personality types. He tried several times to attach a nickname to me—Ben the Monster, Jurassic Ben. None of them ever took. Only in my adult years would I discover that he had considered calling me Tomahawk, which I actually would've liked.

I didn't get along with the guys easily. The girls loved me to pieces, though. Despite there being some hotties, I only ever thought of them as older sisters. I was surprised one day to find that they weren't much older than me, but there was an obvious maturity about them that was greatly lacking in myself. I always saw myself as significantly younger. It never occurred to me to ask any of the girls my age for a date. Only once, toward the end, did I actually consider pursuing a girl, but then I was put off when I discovered her taste in music. I may be too picky.

The only time I felt meaningful in a group was during summer Bible studies, which involved much more interaction than a typical youth group night. Here, my days spent in solitary contemplation had significance for the people around me, and hence, I saw that I mattered. I gained little connection from this, though, because the realization of my spiritual nature caused some to feel inadequate next to me. That didn't occur to me until later.

As I entered adulthood, most of the people I knew from youth group either moved on to other churches or didn't attend the college and career group. Since Anna and Josh had moved away, I felt it was time to look for another church.

At the same time, a friend of the family invited us to Carruthers Creek Community Church (or "C4," as we lovingly call it). My mom and I felt completely at home there.

I attempted their youth group, which I was still welcome to, but still found I couldn't connect. By then, I was practically too old to attend anyway.

I had a bit more success in the small group Bible studies, but only because I was the answer guy. I still fell short when it came to socializing. I was aware that so many other guys my age had lived "the sinful life," wheras I had not, and because of this what was once seen simply as my naivety was now becoming my "innocence" in the eyes of the Christian guys around me—my "purity," my "holiness." Admittedly, I started to think that way, too, and became proud. Even today, I struggle not to look down on people, but I'm at least more aware today that my "innocence" comes from a lack of tempting situations, which most of the guys my age have been subject to in abundance.

After becoming a legal adult, the first phases of teen angst kicked in. I was finally aware of what my life was missing socially, having gone through my high school years without finding any girls to grow up with. Love songs started to take on a new meaning—a depressing meaning. This was a whole new level of feeling inadequate.

I blame *Shrek*. After I saw *A Knight's Tale*, I was definitely put off romance. Having been reminded how indecisive, stupid, and demanding women could be, I felt I could live the rest of my life without them. But when I saw *Shrek*, I was thrown right back into that desire. Probably because it adhered to the Beauty and the Beast kind of romance, which holds more significance for me than the typical love story.

Beauty and the Beast remains one of the most significant movies for my soul, but I can no longer watch it because I'm past my twenty-first year and it hurts too much that I haven't found my Belle.

My issues really started coming out when I joined another Bible study group. This one was an all-guys group approximately my age, all jacked-up on testosterone to the point that trying to speak over the crowd was like a head-butting contest between mountain rams.

I learned more about male social interaction in that one year than in all my previous years, or maybe I was finally ready to connect. It was a completely different atmosphere from the female-dominated household I had grown up in. At home, farts were to be hidden and covered up, or blamed on someone else. Among guys, farts were to be announced and celebrated, and occasionally preluded to. "Here's my opinion..."

The big difference here was the group leader—we'll call him Jacob—who unlike every previous leader I'd been under had a far more liberal approach than I was used to. I was uncomfortable with his ways at first because they were so foreign to me; they allowed guys to be guys with very little observable restraint. Indeed, it was a level of liberalism I wouldn't employ in my own group, yet at the time it was exactly what I needed.

I'm more conservative than liberal by nature. In the church I grew up in, my conservative nature was used against me as a guilt-builder, something to constrain my creative processes. Jacob came from the opposite extreme, with a much stronger understanding of grace. By observing him and his ways, I came to understand the faults of both extremes, and come to a place of balance within myself.

What's more, it was with this group that I was introduced to the writings of John Eldredge, through *Wild at Heart*. That book completely reshaped my perception of what God intended when He made guys, and hence when He made me. It has greatly influenced the progression I've made in recent years.

It was a very dark time in my life when Jacob left, for reasons I was never told. I simultaneously had no small group to attend, a lost leader, and reports of severe struggles going on with everyone else I looked up to. I again felt fatherless, and realized that I had people looking up to me for spiritual direction while I myself had no mentor. If you've never been there, it's a very dark place to be. Even top leaders have counsellors to turn to for answers they cannot find themselves. Nobody is meant to tackle life on their own.

I tried a different small group for a couple of years, a mixed group this time because I needed to learn how to interact with women.

That group didn't work out very well. They had a group-prayer system that forced everyone to pray for the person next to them. I subtly got out of this as often as I could, but sometimes I had to be direct, stating that I was uncomfortable with group prayer. In most groups this would be received with grace, but here it was received with stunned, questioning glances. I contributed in many ways, through answers, thoughts, provocative questions, and suggestions on praise styles. But because of a discomfort with group prayer, I was perceived as uncooperative. I wasn't seen for what I provided, only for what I did not.

Then I joined Alpha, a program for young and old Christians who want to relearn the core beliefs of Christianity. It's also for people who are searching for God and want to see what Christianity has to offer. I finally felt that I had social purpose again, able to answer questions and raise new ones and get people thinking.

Being a part of the Alpha program, I've had the inspiring opportunity to listen to people of various belief systems describe their experiences in life, their views on God, and their questions.

I'm an intellectual thinker, and we tend to simplify a lot of the questions we cannot seem to answer into a matter of faith, training ourselves not to deal with them. But I've determined to take those questions directly to God, in faith that He has answers. Rarely have I walked away without an intellectual answer.

When a person has intellectual reasons for struggling with the idea of God as spoken of in the scriptures, I'm often able to help, or at least understand them, because I have dealt with similar questions.

On the flip side, some of the people who come to Alpha have emotional reasons for struggling with the God we talk about. While I sometimes understand where they're coming from, emotionally, I can detach myself and look at the situation in black and white, seeing the facts as they are. Some people have been thankful to me for this. Others I later realized had deeper emotional struggles than I first thought, and an intellectual answer was the last thing they needed. I'm still learning when my kind of wisdom is needed and when it is not.

These days, I'm striving to understand people's emotions better, while not being dictated by them, so I can both relate to people's pain and help them come to factual solutions. I appear unable to do the same with myself.

CHAPTER FIVE

Interests

In my childhood, I became obsessed with Transformers. I was quite good with them. I didn't even need to read the instructions! Some adults would play with one of my Transformers, unable to figure it out. Then I'd come along, yank it out of their hands, and change it for them.

As soon as my parents started me on Transformers, I wouldn't play with anything else. I would receive a toy and immediately ask what it turned into. I would even take toys that didn't transform and manipulate every single joint until they were something else. I like things that turn into other things, and I have a gift for manipulation and seeing potential for transformation.

I also got heavy into Lego, the ultimate manipulation toy. I had a carrying case that I filled with Lego pieces so I could build robots in my spare time. I liked playing with Lego people and switching their body parts around. When purchasing a Lego set, I still go for the ones with the best characters rather than the most pieces.

DINOSAURS

As a child, my top scientific interest was a tossup between space and dinosaurs. In my younger years, dinosaurs won. I liked creatures more than science itself.

At first, my favourite was probably the T-Rex. But I was aware of the Rex's popularity among other kids; my need to be different from the crowd pushed me to find another dinosaur I liked better. Now it's the Deinonychus, which is kind of like the Velociraptor's evil twin.

My family once let me borrow an illustrated dinosaur book from the church library. It had so many dinosaurs listed with full-page illustrations that it quickly became my favourite book.

At home, I took a marker and drew circles around every dinosaur I wanted to bring into "now-times." I circled the dinosaur and drew a portal with Earth in it. Then I drew lines between the dinosaur and the portal, showing it getting sucked in. I did this for a few pages and then decided I didn't like how the pictures looked with circles drawn on them.

When it came time to give the book back, my family was surprised to see what I had done.

"You can't draw on things that you borrow!" I was told. "They don't belong to you!"

I understood that I would be giving the book back, but apparently I hadn't perceived the consequence. I didn't realize that the circles would still be there when the book was returned.

My family decided to buy the book from the church and let me keep it, but I wasn't allowed to borrow anything else for a long time—not until I showed signs of perceiving consequences.

I still have that book, though it's gradually falling apart from its many years of love. I've gotten a lot of good information out of it.

DRAWING

I was far better at drawing than writing as a child. My obsession with interesting creatures meant that any blank page in a book of mine would soon become home to some strange creature or another. By Grade Two, my obsession switched to Ninja Turtles.

I tended to draw people with their eyeballs popping out of their sockets. This was intended to represent surprise, but most people found it gruesome.

Occasionally I would even draw creatures or people onto already-illustrated pages, either making my art interact with the existing art or making it appear that the existing art was interacting with mine—like drawing a chainsaw-wielding psychotic monster in front of an illustration of someone who looks surprised.

I also drew a lot of pictures of heaven and hell. Of course my own depiction of hell and demons, as a child, was always within the realm of the realities I knew, which was mostly comedy and people getting along with each other through humour. My mother often tried to explain, as much as she could to a child, how unpleasant demons and their abodes actually are. Sometimes my artistic depictions of them would change accordingly, but for the most part I just couldn't comprehend evil—not yet. I spent a long time with the fantasy that, somehow, it was possible for everyone to get along. It would be years before I discovered for myself that some individuals genuinely don't want to get along with others.

I often drew pictures of the kind of video games I wanted to make. But as I got older, it became necessary to explain what certain things were by writing descriptions and background information. Gradually my illustrations became less and less frequent as my writing took up more space on the pages.

STAR WARS

My experience with *Star Wars* is unique. You see, I was still very young when I was first introduced to the *Star Wars* universe. I didn't have any concept of Episodes IV, V, or VI. When I was offered the chance to watch a movie called *Star Wars: Return of the Jedi*, I took it, not having a clue that there had been any part to the story before that.

At the time, *Return of the Jedi* was my entire *Star Wars* universe. Because of that, all the characters were introduced to me in a completely different way than they would have been in either of the other films. Luke Skywalker was not the unlikely hero struggling to become something great; he was already there, having always been a great hero. Leia was not the princess; she was the face behind the bounty hunter. Chewbacca wasn't a cool, beast-like warrior; he was an annoying, whimpering, moaning nuisance. Darth Vader wasn't a despicable villain; he was a lost father. And Han Solo was just a decoration!

My whole perception of these characters was different from everyone else's. Perhaps this is why my approach to fictional characters is different than most. Maybe knowing Darth Vader in that light is the reason I'm partial to fictional villains—out of a hope to see them redeemed.

Sometime later, still in my childhood, I looked for *Star Wars* in the video store, and ended up with an entirely different movie than the one I had expected. Why was there snow instead of a forest? Why was Luke's lightsaber blue? Why didn't Luke know who Yoda was? Why was Luke so surprised that Vader was his father? Eventually I came to realize that this was set before *Return of the Jedi*.

It was even later that I stumbled upon a very strange sight on TV one day. I recognized those characters, but they were doing things I had never seen them do before. What? They were *inside* the Death Star? Luke didn't have the Force? There was a time when Ben didn't glow?

At last my understanding of the *Star Wars* universe came to completion. I now had the full story from beginning to end, and I could make sense of the mess in my head.

At the same time that I got into *Return of the Jedi*, I was also into He-Man. For some reason, I had no *Star Wars* figures, but I had plenty of He-Man toys. I took a bucket I had, drew sharp teeth on the inside of it to look like a Sarlacc Pit, and had the He-Man figures battle on a bridge overlooking it so they'd fall in when they got hit.

My Uncle Rob got me one of those He-Man toys with the chest that flips into a battle-damaged chest when hit. My mother thought it was too graphic and would disturb me. I loved it!

CUT-OUTS

At the age of eight, I began cutting images out of magazines. I would see a character or object I liked and cut around it until I had something that looked like a sticker. At the time, it was about exercising control over my own world by taking existing images and arranging them to my liking—like a create-your-own picture book.

I had a whole drawer full of cut-outs, until one day when I had to rearrange my room. I saw the vast collection of cut-outs, then threw out most of them, keeping only the best ones in bins as memoirs. I still use them from time to time as organizational aid.

I continue to add to my bin of cut-outs whenever I see something I really like. Right now, the bin is a collection of creative images I can go to occasionally for inspiration.

I recall setting up clusters of cut-outs according to a story, for the purpose of knowing where certain characters were at any one time. When holding a cut-out in my hand and deciding where it should go, or just thinking in general, I would spin the paper between my thumb and forefinger. I think this was just a deep-thought motion, like clicking a pen or chewing gum.

It may have started when I would take two cut-outs in my hands and imagine the battle between the two represented characters, but however it started, it eventually became just another physical expression of thought.

WRITING

Writing eventually became my main tool for expressing ideas. It wasn't enough for me to just visualize the characters; a need grew in me to keep records of character history, where they came from, and the possibilities of where they might go. The game *Mortal Kombat* inspired this. The incentive of the game was that if you won with a certain character, you got to learn more about their background, or you got to see what happened to them in the future. I found that very intriguing.

By the time I'd played *Turok* and *GoldenEye 007*, I was imagining entire worlds and races with their own intertwining histories. The line between writing stories for movies and writing stories for video games started to blur.

STATS

I have an addiction to stats, facts, and other info—the kind of info most people wouldn't care about. The same way that baseball fans obsess over the stats of each player, updating them after every game, I have an obsession with video game character stats.

Part of it is probably the desire to keep my imaginary tournaments as accurate as possible. I'm also interested in history. I enjoy shows like *Weaponology*, which show you how a certain weapon concept progressed from its earliest form to the form it has today—for example, the progression from a Gatling Gun to a Tommy Gun to an MP7. I like to see things progress.

CREATURES

As a child, I liked creatures more than people. When asked what I wanted to be when I grew up, I would have to give a reasonable answer, but what I really wanted was to be some kind of reptilian creature.

When a video game gave me a choice of what character to play as, my favourite was always the most unique character, the one that looked least human. *Killer Instinct* had my favourite character roster of all time because so few of the characters looked human.

It wasn't until my teen years that I began to identify better with the human characters—in particular, the ones who looked like they'd been around a while and had endured a lot of battles. Whether human or not, the scarred characters were the ones most likely to be living out their existence to its fullest extent—the most honourable ones.

The veteran types are still my favourites, the ones I identify with and admire most. I also favour powerful and ranged characters, as opposed to the fast or defensive.

FAVOURITE CHARACTERS

My top favourite fictional characters of all time are all villains. For some reason, I've always favoured the villains on kids shows. I don't like the bad things villains do, but I find that in most things the villains are a hundred times cooler than the good guys. I see this as a horrendous misrepresentation of the forces of good. Why are the good guys always so lame and boring while the villains have awesome armblades and pet monsters?

Since *Teenage Mutant Ninja Turtles* was my favourite show, my favourite villain was Shredder. Shredder was a unique villain because he was a completely natural human in a show that was all about mutants.

56

He had no mutation and no super powers. He was armed only with what a man can do. I once saw him beat each of the Ninja Turtles using his fighting skills alone. That, by the way, was also the first time I ever realized good guys could lose a fight!

I never liked watching the villains die. I was alright with them going to jail so they could smarten up, but I hated anybody dying.

Three of my favourite characters are Mewtwo, Venom, and T-1000, and each of them are variations or upgrades of other characters. Mewtwo, from *Pokémon*, is a genetically altered copy of Mew; Venom is a cooler looking, more powerful version of Spider-Man, and the T-1000 is the successor to the T-101 model from the first *Terminator* movie. What does that say about myself? Perhaps that I like being similar but unique to the norm, I like the idea of improving on what's already there.

The best example of my kind of character is Beta-Ray Bill from the Thor comics. I don't read comics, but I found Bill's bio on a website and it's the perfect story for a guy like me.

Thor, the main character and ultra-powerful hero, misplaces his hammer one day, which is the source of his power. A freaky horse-faced alien from a fire planet shows up and picks up Thor's hammer, taking all of Thor's powers, including his Norse god armour, and becoming Beta-Ray Bill. Thor complains to his father, Odin, about losing his power and Odin arranges for a contest, a fair fight between Thor and Beta-Ray Bill for ownership of the hammer.

Bill wins.

Then Odin decides to give Thor his old hammer back, but also makes one of equal power called Storm Breaker to give to Bill. Isn't that interesting? Thor must've been thinking nobody could beat him, because he was the original hero, but then he had his butt handed to him by some random freak who just happened to show up while Thor was being irresponsible—and Odin honours this by allowing the new guy to keep his own version of the same power.

So now there's this freaky red horse-faced guy walking around in Norse god armour (with the winged helmet and everything) flying around smashing stuff with a hammer equivalent to the power of Thor. That's so beautiful!

Comic books seem like the kind of thing I should like, but I was never able to get into them. Comic books have an element of raw fantasy and escapism that I usually go for, but there's something about still images that bother me—a single moment frozen in time, never to change. If it's an image of suffering, it might trigger my perception of hell. Certain repetitive music types have a similar effect on me.

CHAPTER SIX

Video Game Interaction

Video games have always been a favourite hobby of mine. They provided an escape, a way of interacting with someone else's world. Rather than movies, in which you are told what happens and you have to sit there and accept it, video games allow you to decide the outcome and events taking place during the story.

In *Tetris*, I intentionally put pieces in the most awkward locations until they take up half the screen, then I try playing properly, bringing order to chaos.

My mother noticed, before I did, that I had a gift for manipulating games. I would observe how certain aspects of the game affected each other and use that to my advantage, or entertainment. For instance, in *GoldenEye 007*, I set up motion-sensing mines in bathroom stalls so they would explode whenever someone needed to go.

The best video games for me are the ones that let you create, customize, and envision. These provide a way for me to truly express myself. It took too long for video games to reach that point, and then only a few integrated that concept. Customizing is becoming more and more common in video games today, to the extent that the average gamer can design not only their own characters, but vehicles, levels, buildings, race tracks, and weapons as well.

As a teen, video games were the easiest way for me to connect with other people—partly because they brought both me and the other person into the same world, making us equals, but also because they were the best way for me to express myself. Video games allowed me to create, manipulate, and customize.

No two people play the same game the exact same way, and any change in my own approach to a classic game reveals changes within myself. It is easy to develop a routine once you're good at a game. Any deviation from that routine can be a sign of inner growth.

Lego Star Wars is one of my favourite video game franchises. It's accessible to so many more people than the average game, it provides a variety of characters to choose from, and it encourages cooperative play. The reason I enjoy it so much is that I can play it with just about anybody. Anyone can play their own way while at the same time interacting with me the way I play.

There was a time when video games were the only way I could interact with people and be myself. This was a challenge since neither of my parents were into video games, at least not until I was old enough to socialize in other ways. Add to that the fact that I had very few friends, and you'll see that I almost never interacted with people the way I did best.

My sisters played at first, but they grew out of it. Nonetheless, they enjoyed watching me play because it was like an art for me, or a sport. I would get so good at a game that my method for a level became as much an act of precision as archery. I suppose that's the repetitive and monotonous aspect of my autism, but it works pretty well. I'm especially annoying to play against in racing games once I've practiced the courses.

RPGs

I like upgrades. I like when things improve. I like when I improve. I like seeing the process of one thing becoming something else. I like to observe progression. This is probably why Role-Playing Games (RPGs) are especially attractive to me, as is any game where you start off with almost nothing and work your way up to becoming the most powerful force in the game.

Lately, I've taken to researching every move a Pokémon can learn, how it learns it, and which top moves it needs to be ideal for my team.

Then I look at what ways the Pokémon will need to be raised in order to have all those moves. I like seeing the maximum potential of something and figuring out strategies to bring out its full potential.

And since I have a gift for organizing, managing an inventory is a lot of fun for me—sometimes more fun than the gameplay itself.

I like arranging teams. That sounds odd, since I have difficulty functioning on teams in real life, but I like figuring out ways of putting the strengths of each character to use in such a way that the entire team functions as one strong unit.

Some people have the mindset that if you're weak in one area, that's the area you need to focus on strengthening. This strategy may be best if you're working alone, but on a team each person should focus on doing what they are especially gifted at. If you aren't good at one thing, chances are someone else on the team can do it instead. You focus on your own areas of strength; you may be the only one who can do what you can do.

Getting everyone to work on improving the areas in which they are weak results in wasted time, neglected strengths, and a team where everyone is the same. There may be no weaknesses, but neither are there strengths.

I think my interest in how individuals with unique strengths operate on a team is one of my ways of trying to see where I fit into the world. It's important for me to know that something I've done has actually had a positive impact on those around me. Most of the time I feel like it wouldn't matter to those around me whether or not I was present.

I often look at teams of fictional characters and ask the people I know, "Which one of those people am I most like?" Most people can look at a group of fictional characters and spot which is most like their friend; some can even spot themselves. I cannot. Shanks always sees me as the wise one in a group—Gandalf, Qui-Gon Jinn, or Morpheus. He sees me as the good teacher. I know this is mainly because I've been more of a mentor to him than anything else.

Other than Shanks, when I ask this kind of question, I rarely get an answer. Partly this may be because it's hard for others to recognize my intellect. Once I entered my mid-twenties, though, people were more willing to accept my gifts. As a teenager, however, my wisdom was rarely recognized.

Well, I've come to understand that a big reason that I haven't found my place in the community is that the community has disregarded the part I've always been meant to play. The Bible says, *"Don't let anyone look down on you because you are young, but set an example for the believers in speech, in life, in love, in faith and in purity"* (1 Timothy 4:12). I believe this is also the reason for compulsive organization, such as we see in little children lining up small objects in a specific order, and me with Pokémon cards.

In her book, *Nobody Nowhere*, Donna Williams, a high-functioning autistic says about her beloved collection of buttons, ribbons, sequins and coloured tinfoil and glass:

> I could lay everything out in categories and grasp the concept of order, consistency, and belonging despite my inner lack of it. I could see what role each thing had in relation to the next, unlike my relationships with people. Unlike my life, all my special things had their own undeniable place within the scheme of things… When I set out my bits and pieces, I could visually grasp the elusive sense of belonging I could never feel with people, and through this could give myself hope that it would one day be possible. I could see it, laid out in front of me in categories of things that could be arranged slowly and gently to blend into one another in some concrete, observable, and totally orderly way.[1]

ISSUES WITH VIDEO GAMES

Video games were once a dangerous point of frustration for me. I was about eight before my mother thought it okay for me to have a game system. Even then, I would get mad and stomp up the stairs when things didn't go as I wanted them to.

My mother removed the game whenever I acted up. This helped

---

[1] Donna Williams, *Nobody Nowhere* (New York, NY: Doubleday), 1992, 163.

me understand how to maintain control over the game. If I got to the point that I was getting frustrated and acting up, the game would be removed. I learned to stick to the places in the game where I wouldn't be frustrated. If the entire game was frustrating, I learned that it wasn't worth playing.

The problem was obsession and single-mindedness. Once I had my mind on a task, it was next to impossible to think about anything else until that task was done.

Games don't frustrate me quite so much anymore. I can't pinpoint an exact time when I stopped having tantrums over them. I would say that it's been a gradual growth process.

I have had tantrums over other things—pretty much all having to do with technology. I realize now that one of the most frustrating things for me is when something doesn't do what it's programmed to do. I once wrote a blog post that went something like this:

Have you ever had one of those moments when you tell a computer to do something and it doesn't do that? In fact, it sends you a message stating that it can't do that, but you know full well it *can* do that. Because you've seen it do that before. Why is it just choosing not to do that now?

I had a printer, and I told the printer to print something, and it sent me a message stating, in summary, "I can't do that."

I thought, "Well, why did I buy you?"

If something says "printer" on it, and it can't print, isn't that false advertising?

Sometimes my computer tells me it can't do something, but I know full well it can, so I repeat the command. Sometimes I have to repeat the command several times, but eventually it does the thing I commanded it to do. It's like it just forgot that it could do that and it had to be told a specific number of times before it would remember.

"I can't do that."

"I can't do that."

"I can't do that."

"Oh, wait—I *can* do that."

Isn't it frustrating when something doesn't do what it's told to do, especially when you know it's the very thing it was created to do?

I have to sympathize with God here. He made each of us for a specific purpose, something we are fully equipped to do, something that is the very reason for our being—and we refuse to do it. Sometimes we feel the need to inform God, "I can't do that," since He obviously doesn't know what we were made for.

God gave us free will, so it's expected that we will do whatever we choose to do with ourselves. Except I don't recall giving my printer free will.

You will never be more fulfilled than when you live your life according to what God designed you specifically to do. If you ignore His prompts, He's gonna keep reminding you all your life, until you do what you've been called to do. If you fight your very purpose for being, you'll be as useful as a printer that doesn't print.

Have you ever created something for a specific purpose and been annoyed when it didn't work? Have you ever felt the pride of seeing something you've created perform the task you made it for?

Whatever quirks you may have, whatever issues some people may have with the real you, when you walk, talk, act, and think the way God personally made you to, God looks on you with delight and says, "Look at that! I made that!"

I hate time limits. I hate having to do a certain thing within a certain amount of time. My brain takes longer to work than most people, but the results are highly inventive. Having to compromise my usual thought process for a timer is very stressful and frustrating. I even have trouble conversing with fast-paced people because they demand immediate answers to their questions. My only defence is, "Be patient. My words are worth the wait."

It's probably why I'm so stressed about life, worrying about getting everything done, when I don't even know everything I'm supposed to do.

I've concluded that my dislike of time limits is part of the way I've been wired for Eden. God has set eternity in my heart. I wasn't meant to live in a world with a time limit.

I don't mind beating a video game level within a time limit to unlock something. That teaches time management. But I don't like a timer being an essential and inescapable part of the gameplay.

MAZES

As a child, I really, *really* liked mazes. I was obsessed with them. I also used to draw mazes—everywhere—and then solve my own mazes. I was given a book of dinosaur mazes and then had to draw my own as well, only to solve them.

I had a schoolbook called "My Friend the Policeman" and on the notes section on the back, I drew a maze.

I think it was the sense of journey combined with problem solving. If one path didn't work, I could take another path. I enjoyed figuring out how to get from here to there.

People around me considered drawing mazes a talent. Perhaps they still do. I didn't actually need to have the entire thing planned out from the beginning; I knew how to draw mazes as an art, without worrying about whether or not the path connected from point A to point B. I could even completely lose track of where the path was as I drew the maze.

The trick is to draw the walls as you would a bizarre tree. You might start just drawing the trunk, having it turn and curve and zigzag depending on the style of your art. It's actually quite expressive. From there, you can add branches, curving and zigzagging next to and around existing lines. You can start as many trees and branches as you like, sprouting from the edges of the maze or even starting in open space if you prefer, continuing on until you have only thin corridors.

The only rule is that no branches can touch each other, so as to make a dead end. Plenty of dead ends can be made by sprouting branches that keep close to an existing wall, before traveling further off. The trick to making sure the path remains, without having to keep track of the path as you draw, is to make sure no branches meet. The result is a maze where even you don't know the right path. It's your own creation and yet you have to figure it out just like everyone else.

CHAPTER SEVEN

Struggles

A.D.D.

I still struggle in church when the congregation listens to one person pray. In my childhood, I didn't know exactly what this was about. *Do I just listen? Am I supposed to repeat it in my mind? What happens if I don't listen properly?* I would think all this while the guy was praying, and get very little out of what was said.

Although I don't worry or beat myself up as much these days, I still struggle to listen. This is also true of group prayer. While people speak of the issues they're having, it's an unfortunate truth that I can only listen to so much before my mind gets caught on a single subject. If it's one of those groups where everyone has to pray, and you don't get to pick who you pray for, I'm screwed. This is why I avoid groups that force prayer onto people. It's always been difficult for me to include other people in what I consider to be very personal time with my Saviour. I also pray much better on my own without the threat of time limits.

DESTRUCTIVE BEHAVIOUR

Tantrums were common in my childhood. They were typically the result of my frustration over not knowing how to communicate my needs. I've even destroyed things that were valuable to me, out of pure rage. In my teen years, tantrums became a rare occurrence. In my adult life, they've been pretty much absent but for one relapse a few years ago involving an uncooperative ceiling fan.

If you were to come over to my house, you'd see that I have a drawer missing from my dresser. A day came when I needed to direct my frustration toward something not very valuable, and the drawer got the short straw. I could get a new dresser, so that I don't have that empty space, a reminder of the time my strength failed, but oddly it doesn't remind me so much of my shortcoming but of God's forgiveness. I've never looked at it as a negative reminder.

Although I may get a new dresser when I start running out of space for clothes.

I only remember biting myself once, as a kid, and not to the point of drawing blood. I don't know if I made a habit out of it, because I only remember doing it the one time. It was out of frustration, mostly at my circumstances. I don't even remember what the circumstances were—I only remember how I felt.

So, why bite myself? There's no logical reason. I just felt that something had to suffer, something had to be punished—not necessarily me, but I wouldn't hurt anyone else.

Once while at Dunder Mifflin, I attempted suicide using a pencil. Apparently I wasn't sane enough at the time to differentiate between the sharp end and the rubber end. I wonder now if my logic at the time was to erase myself.

POOR EATING HABITS

Through research, I discovered that gastrointestinal problems are quite common for people with Asperger's. At the same time, I learned that atypical eating (specifically, eating too much of the same food) is also quite common. I wasn't sure if the intestinal problems were a direct side effect of Asperger's or a direct result of atypical eating, so I consulted my doctor and he confirmed that the latter was most likely the case.

Atypical eating is one of many behavioural dysfunctions with the same root—a need for sameness. A need for unwavering routine. Sameness equals security.

Hot dogs were my staple food for several years. I ate three hot dogs almost every day, except when leftover pizza was available. My mother always cooked healthy dinners when she got home from work, while during the day I enjoyed solitude at home, working on my writing and making my own meals. She always told me it was unhealthy to eat too many hot dogs, but I didn't see the problem until I noticed a change in my well-being.

Another eating problem was connected to all my microwavable lunches. Microwave radiation kills so many important nutrients. That's when I realized I needed to learn to cook using the stove. I'm still learning simple things like pizza and stew, things that don't require me to time multiple objects at once, since I can't multitask. I've just perfected Kraft Dinner.

Yet another problem I've run into is that every time I make an effort to try something new, and like it, I end up only wanting that thing. Getting out of these behavioural eating patterns requires continual variety and balance.

I'm an advocate for balance, but I don't manage it very well.

Another thing I've been told to do is eat smaller meals, more frequently. Actually, my body already got to the point that it didn't want to eat large meals anymore; I've been that way for a while, but I didn't know I'd have to eat more often throughout the day. Generally every two hours or so I should have something, even if only a snack. It's recommended that I have the traditional three meals a day, lighter than usual, with even lighter meals between breakfast and lunch, and then again between lunch and dinner.

I'm starting to feel like a hobbit—breakfast, second breakfast, elevensies, luncheon, afternoon tea, dinner, and supper. For a guy who has to learn to eat less, I feel like I'm pigging out.

Ideally, I need more balanced eating habits. I haven't figured out how to manage this, since it requires a drastic change in habits and self-discipline. At least I know that it's not an automatic result of Asperger's. As a behavioural problem, it can be overcome with work.

SLEEPING

I also found out in my research that sleep disorders are very common for people with Asperger's. Although my research didn't bring up the exact nature of the disorders, I have struggled with sleeping problems for a while now.

At first it was not a major problem; I just worked on a slightly different schedule than most people. I think some people with later sleeping schedules are necessary for the world to work. I call it the Theory of the Night Watchman. In the tribal era of our species, when it was necessary for someone to be watching the borders at all times, we adapted by producing a few rare individuals with a natural tendency to function better in the evening and night times, as opposed to the morning or afternoon like the average person, thus providing a full circulation of guards around the clock, each one serving when they're at their best.

I think this is the case with me. I am *not* a morning a person.

Even though I seem to be better off getting up a bit later in the morning and getting to sleep late at night, my current sleeping schedule is so drastic that I'm sleeping into the afternoon most days. I know part of the reason is interrupted sleep, but there's got to be something more to it that I'm missing.

People have advised me that it's a simple matter of getting to bed sooner, as if that idea had not occurred to me. I find that going to bed when I'm not tired is the worst possible thing for me to do. I don't have an on-and-off switch as some people apparently have. If I get into bed and I'm not tired, all I'll succeed in doing is lying there for hours, spending no energy at all, getting frustrated for not falling asleep. It results in me getting to sleep much later than I would have if I had stayed up until I knew I was tired enough to fall asleep.

I think what it comes down to is that I need to exercise more during the day and get out more for some fresh-air walks. My backyard is a forest, so I have the perfect home for pacing around outside.

Society demands that I sleep at certain hours for a certain length of time and get up and have enough energy for the day. Since this doesn't work for me, it's just one of many reasons this world doesn't feel right for me. God knows what He's doing, but I have to ask what the heck He was doing when He put a person like me in a world like this.

I hate that our lifespans are so short. Time limits are so much of a burden for me. It's not as if I can't get things done; I just can't get things done within the allotted time. And if I try to do things at my own pace, people tell me I'm too slow or too lazy.

I don't necessarily think I need more hours in the day, but I would prefer if I had the freedom to sleep when I was tired and wake up when I'm refreshed, which would require more than twenty-four hours. This would mean stretching my days so that I have six "days" (or six "sleeps") in the course of a week. I say, let everyone follow their own day/night system and I'll follow my tired/energized system. I'd be fine with that, but everyone around me feels neglected.

Theoretically, an autistic needs a daily pattern in order to function properly. Maybe I do, too. If I could only be permitted to sleep when I'm tired, get up when I'm refreshed, and eat when I'm hungry, I might fall into a pattern of my own that works. God doesn't work according to my pattern, however, and the Sunday church service starts at ten o'clock in the morning whether I'm tired or not. And those social meetings at church are too important to me to set aside for sleep.

I have to be more careful about eating late at night because of heartburn. To combat this, I force myself not to sleep until at least three hours after a meal, which is very difficult.

For a time, my church had an extra service at night targeted toward young adults, and I was finally able to attend a church sermon while at my most awake. I hoped to make connections with others my age and get a sense of what the people of my generation were doing, how they were living—I've been disconnected for so long—but it eventually shifted from a young adults ministry to a youth ministry, and I couldn't connect with anyone or follow the message very well.

THE INFINITE

The concept of infinity has bothered me since an early age, when I was told there was no end to space and that God had no beginning, that heaven would never end. My mind doesn't work in infinites; it works in containment. Any concept that demands to be outside that containment cannot be.

Some people simply accept these things on faith, but as a child I couldn't accept anything outside my understanding. I could understand that God created the universe. All that required was a big imagination. But an infinite universe? That's incomprehensible. And if something's incomprehensible, it cannot be maintained and cannot exist.

Most kids might hear of these things and say, "Whoa!" But in my case this would result in panic attacks. Anytime I tried to grasp something I knew couldn't be contained in my mind, I would fall to the floor and scream. A part of me wanted heaven to end one day just so I wouldn't have to think about it.

One time at South Park, I wanted to draw the universe as it was before God created it. But if God hadn't created it yet, what colour was it? I freaked out and started screaming in the classroom.

The teachers got my mother on the phone and forced me to talk to her. I somehow explained what I was trying to do and that I couldn't figure it out. My mother said, "Black."

I went back to my desk and resumed drawing, quiet and calm.

FACIAL RECOGNITION

I'm much better at this today, but in my childhood, as with most people with autism, telling one person from another was a great challenge.

Because my two sisters are so close together in age, and they both had long hair, for a long time I called them both "Anna." That is, until one day my younger sister shouted, "For the fifty-millionth time, my name is *Karen*!" So I called them both "Karen." After a while of that, I heard, "Actually, my name is Anna." At which point I probably gave up, wishing she'd make up her mind.

Women, honestly!

SECURITY

Remember the game I made up to play with my neighbourhood friends, "Be Whoever You Want to Be"? Well, the most important thing for me was the establishment of bases—your character's home. I had to know that my base was secure enough that the other characters couldn't break in before I was ready. I had to know that I was safe until I decided to fight, and could then go out and seek battle on my terms. This wasn't for the sake of relaxing securely in my base all day, although I liked to know I had that option; it was important to me that my base, though acknowledged as imaginary, was a safe place.

Clearly this was more important to me than I would've thought, as proven one day when I was playing one-on-one with a kid who refused to let my base be a safe place. No matter what kind of security I set up, he invented some reason why he could still get in, even past the point of being reasonable.

At a wiser age, I would have simply walked away, explaining why I wasn't having fun playing with him. But we were both stubborn and immature and something inside me snapped. I don't remember if I screamed or shouted, but I very insistently said, "No!" I froze in place, staring into nothing in particular. The kid continued to say something I didn't care enough to listen to; I perceived only that he was still trying to get his way. All I could say was "No." That was my only response to anything he said after that. Eventually he left.

I stayed in that position, staring with indignant rage at nothing in particular, when the kid came back and said his mom said he could break into my base. Obviously I countered with, "No." The kid left.

I don't remember what did or didn't happen after that, but I understood that if I wasn't going to play by this kid's rules, I would eventually have to leave his backyard. It was just unfortunate that this had been the spot where I broke down. Having had what any perceptive person would see as a psychotic episode, it was difficult for me to move so much as my eyes off whatever I had been staring at so hatefully.

I did eventually make it back to my place. I don't know if word got out or if the other kids were wiser, but that incident never repeated itself.

Reading this over, I'm surprised the boy didn't know I was having a breakdown. Maybe by then he had already seen me being "odd," so this was nothing new to him. Or maybe he'd dealt with other kids' tantrums and didn't see this as being any different. I suppose I should be thankful I wasn't treated differently at the time.

EYE CONTACT

Why the struggle with eye contact? For most people, the reluctance to make eye contact stems from a fear of being figured out, a fear of people seeing the evil within us. Eye contact creates a kind of nakedness. People can see inside you when you make eye contact. Guilt-ridden people struggle with eye contact a lot. Avoiding eye contact is a way of covering up.

I don't know if autistics typically suffer from guilt to a greater extent than most people. I do know that I struggled a lot with guilt, to the extent that as an adult I still felt guilty for the problems I may have caused as a child. Thank God I'm past that now.

Some have observed that an autistic may talk more openly while riding in the car. This is because while riding in a car the expectation is to look forward or out the window, not at each other. The pressure to make eye contact is removed and everyone is free to look wherever they choose and communicate verbally without the forced atmosphere of nakedness that eye contact creates.

I've heard it said that eye contact avoidance is common of guys in general, not just autistics, though the switch between introversion and extroversion in and out of the car is probably more extreme with autistic guys. I don't know if it's the same with autistic women.

I was in my teens when I first recognized that all my little habits pointed to a fear of getting in the way, of being an interference, of causing more problems than I solved. I saw it in my behaviour in public places, like grocery stores—my primary objective was not to get as much done as possible but instead to get in the way as little as possible, to waste as little time as possible, to interfere as little as possible.

These thoughts may have been placed on me by others, or by myself in worrying about what others thought of me. I was aware that I was a problem, in many cases. I didn't create as many problems in my later childhood, but I felt fully responsible for any problems I created when I was younger.

Eventually, I developed this saying: "It is because of me, but it is not my fault." I had to recognize that I hadn't chosen to be autistic. It had been forced upon me. In my mind, you were only at fault if the problem was caused by your decision, not your existence.

I struggled for so long because the feeling kept coming back that my life was screwed up, that I was hopeless, and that I had made myself this way. At the age of twenty-four, I could finally articulate my reasoning this way: *You are not responsible for your circumstances, only how you respond to them.*

Perfectionism

I constantly battle perfectionism, the feeling that I should be doing better, that I ought to know better. Learning how to improve isn't good enough—I should have *already* known what to do. This is a very unhealthy mindset. In response to this way of thinking, I've learned to say to myself, "Don't look at it as one more thing you're doing wrong. Look at it as encouragement that it's one more way in which you're ready to improve."

Perfectionism in general is a need to be good for something. Many people aren't quite sure what they need to be perfect for; they just know that they need to. When growing up in the church, the "cause" for perfection is specific—to please God.

Actually, in my case I already understood that God accepted me as I was, because the suffering of Jesus paid the price for all my iniquities (my intentional sins, not my genetic issues). My perfectionism was not about ensuring my place in heaven, because I already knew I was going there no matter what. My perfectionism was the manifestation of a need I felt to make up for my sins, to make up for the suffering Jesus had to go through.

I was shocked when I finally realized this. Isn't this the kind of self-destructive thinking that Jesus died to remove? By trying to make up for Jesus' suffering on the cross for my sins, am I not in actuality trying to make up for my sins directly? Am I not trying to *earn* my place in heaven? The night I realized this, I felt the Lord speak to me: "I died for *all* your sins. Stop trying to take that away from me. You have to give me all of it."

75

I confessed what I had unconsciously been trying to do all those years, and I gave it all to Him. Finally realizing what accepting Christ's atonement meant was a major struggle. It meant giving up the right to say, "I atoned for all my own sins. I have justified myself. I earned my place in heaven." My man-genes kicked into gear at the thought of that. Is it right to accept someone else's sacrifice to make up for your own screw-ups? I didn't think so. It seemed like taking my sins on my own shoulders was the honourable thing to do, even if it resulted in damnation.

Then I realized that the essence of heaven isn't eternal happiness—it's fellowship with God. It is to be in God's presence for eternity, which happiness is simply a direct result of. By wanting to earn my place in heaven, I'm saying to God, "I don't want to be with you for eternity unless I earn my place there. And if I don't make it, I'll gladly take damnation instead, as long as I get what I deserve. That's the important thing."

That sounds perfectly honourable. So what's wrong with this mindset? God doesn't care that I earn my place with Him, obviously, or else He wouldn't have gone through the excruciation of the cross to atone for me. That's not to say God doesn't have a sense of justice. In fact, His holy justice is why the cross was necessary; *somebody* had to atone for the evils of the world. That I justify my own existence is not important to God—He created me, He obviously feels that my creation was just.

What matters to God is that I am with Him, forever. He suffered and died on the cross so that we could be together. It is not my place to tell God that He should care more about my honour than my salvation. What matters to Him is what brings Him honour. I bring Him honour by admitting that I don't deserve to be in His presence, and by acknowledging that even if I did live a perfect life, I would never be worthy of His presence. This life is not a qualifying exam—it's a rehearsal.

I view going to the dentist the way most people view going to church. He's just going to examine, criticize, and condemn. He won't see or appreciate any of the effort I've made; he only points out what

I've done wrong. He never gives me any tangible advice on how to do better. Instead I get extreme commands like, "Never drink pop again" or "Never eat cereal." His advice is only for perfection and nothing short of it; there's no effort to meet me halfway. It's uncomfortable, it's exposing, it's condemning, and I'll only be made to feel bad for going. But if I don't want an eternity of suffering, what choice do I have?

Thank God I found a supportive church that doesn't feel like going to the dentist!

It was a long time before I could lose while playing a video game and realize that it was okay. These days, I'm wise enough to recognize that a lot of the difficulty in video games comes from incompetent programmers. But even when I lose on a game that's properly made, I handle it better than I did as a kid. I can still get obsessive and play for ages until I beat it, but I'm no longer emotional or prone to tantrums over games.

THE TWO LOVES

The following is an excerpt from my personal journal.

March 13, 2009

Having a mother and father to raise you provides you with two important aspects of love and teaches you how to recognize and receive that love from God as you develop.

Growing up with a distant father and an attentive mother and older sisters, I received an abundant dose of the nurturing kind of love, the kind that lets me know I'll be okay if I fall. But I received none of the love that encourages me to do better. I don't know what that love feels like or how to recognize it.

Anytime I'm told I should do better, it's accompanied with a feeling that I can't pull it off, that it's beyond me and I'm hopeless. Fatherly love doesn't force on you a sense of obligation that you should do better, but encourages you that you can and will do better.

Since nurturing love is the only love I know, I fear I've become over dependant on it. I don't have the encouraging love that's so desperately needed to balance it out. Knowing that I'm unconditionally accepted, I'm easily enticed to not even try to do better.

Aware of this danger, I try to avoid that pit by stepping away from the nurturing love, and end up overcompensating. Without knowing what the other love looks like, I move away from one love but don't find another. I don't find the balance I need. Instead of shifting focus from one love to another, in an attempt to balance I reject one and allow no love at all—until I fall and find myself needing to be nurtured again. Lacking fatherly love, I've developed a self-drivenness which, coupled with my fear of overdependence on nurturing love, creates a hopeless, unholy striving.

Typically I'm not an emotional person, but there have been times in recent years when I've suddenly been overcome by powerful emotions that take me a minute to identify. One time was when I was with family and was struck by the emotion of gratitude. Apparently I hadn't been feeling it often enough, but when I saw my family together in harmony I was overcome by this emotion I didn't immediately know the name of.

Twice I've been hit by an overwhelming sense of being loved. Both times have been when I was struggling to decide what was the right thing to do in a situation and was praying desperately for guidance. I desired to please God, but I didn't know which decision would please Him and which would make Him angry. He then reminded me that He loved me and would continue to love me no matter what decision I made, and also that He knew my heart and the earnestness with which I prayed to Him.

THE BLAME AND GUILT MENTALITY

Growing up, I was harshly affected by a mentality of blame and guilt. Whenever something went wrong, you had to find someone to blame, and then heap on the guilt for whatever went wrong. Mistakes couldn't just be forgotten; they had to be embedded into your psyche.

Whenever anything went wrong, you had to quickly find someone to put the blame on. If the blame fell on you, you would try hard to shift it onto someone else. Whoever the blame ultimately fell on would never hear the end of it.

This led to a fear of making decisions, because if anything went wrong, the blame would be placed on whoever made the decision. I feared making mistakes, so I also feared changing anything or trying anything new. A group of us couldn't try something new and laugh when it didn't work out; we would blame whoever's idea it was and never let them forget it.

Such a mentality also causes people to be overly defensive. People who have suffered from an environment of blame and guilt will defend themselves aggressively to make sure no more blame falls on them.

When anything goes even slightly wrong, even if someone else willingly accepts the blame, an overly defensive person will continue to press blame on anyone other than themselves. They'll defend themselves to the point of offending others, thinking they're only trying to protect themselves.

In recent years, I've fought long and hard to get rid of this mentality. And I succeeded. The blame and guilt mentality has been replaced by one of grace. I've given myself permission to make mistakes. When something goes wrong, I don't rush to place the blame; I rush to solve the problem. I give others permission to make mistakes and learn from them.

I didn't realize how far I'd come from that mentality until I visited another household and saw the mentality there. To the extent that I felt it being pressed on me, that they wouldn't grant me permission to make mistakes, I pressed back with my new approach, continuing to do things with an attitude of grace. It was sad to see, but it made me realize the kind of crap I had gotten out of and how far away from it I'd come.

These days, I recognize it where I wouldn't have when I was still trapped in that mentality. Now that I know what I've come out of, I see it far more vividly in the people around me.

CRITICISM

I don't handle criticism well. I find that most of the negative criticism I get is a result of being misunderstood. Writing is easy; letting people read it is hard.

I've always desired to be understood, for people to realize why I am the way that I am and not judge my conduct against the conduct of a person with different motives than me. I find people judge me too often by lumping me together with people who have a different set of problems than I do.

The worst is when people pass quick and hard judgement about my actions without asking me about it first. Quite often people take a simple misunderstanding and blow it up into a lecture on ethics.

I struggle with gullibility. I probably wouldn't listen to people's opinions as often if I better understood that people are generally as lost as I am. I have head knowledge of that, but not applied knowledge. If I could get to that point of realizing that nobody has everything figured out, I might not take criticism so hard.

Another reason I don't take criticism well, which is also why I need constant encouragement, is that I'm starved for acceptance. Throughout my childhood, people questioned my conduct, telling me I should be different. That continued in my teenage years, then on into my twenties. People haven't let up on me. Everybody feels I should be doing this or that, only it never comes across as encouragement; it comes across as judgement.

Essentially, my struggle with criticism is the result of a failure to comprehend the love of God. I hear it every Sunday: "No one can fathom the love of God." So I never bothered to try. That itself is a contradiction to my usual logic, because although I know it's impossible for me to know everything about God, I still strive to know as much as I can. That's the whole point. It's like when you've been married to someone for fifty years and continue to learn new things about them everyday. Discovering God isn't a one-time event; it's a never-ending adventure.

If I had a better comprehension of God's love for me, I wouldn't worry so much about getting and maintaining the acceptance of others.

In my notes from a recent Bible study, I wrote, "People often criticize in others what they see in themselves." This didn't occur to me because I was being judged by other members of the group, but because I found myself judging them, realized I was doing it quite often, and asked myself why.

I can be a very critical person—especially when watching TV commercials. When I criticize the conduct of other people—or the writing of a book, movie, or TV show—it's often because I'm worried that I make those same mistakes. By thinking about what the person is doing wrong, I'm actually giving myself instructions on how to avoid doing the same thing, but without feeling like I'm disciplining myself because the advice is directed outwardly instead of inwardly. Of course, I've caught on to this now, so hopefully next time I feel like criticizing someone I'll remember to take it as advice that I'm giving to myself.

ANXIETY

After doing some research, I've discovered that anxiety, stress, and depression are quite common for high-functioning autistics. We have no visual signs of mental challenges, and we're average enough for most people to have no idea there's anything different about us. Thus, expectations are put on us to function on all levels at least as well as anyone else.

I don't know how many high-functioning autistics battle with perfectionism, but I have done so all my life. Because we are so much like everyone else, we expect a lot of ourselves, and we put ourselves down when we don't match up. The problem is, I can't always differentiate between what humans expect of me (including myself) and what God expects of me. Nobody knows—even I don't know—what my limits are and what standards I should have. Only God does. Too often, pride and honour goad me into pushing myself up to the world's standards. I should focus less on my honour and focus on honouring God by using what I have for His purposes.

People who struggle with perfectionism to the extent that I do will question the benefit of staying in this world. People who get angry and disappointed with themselves every time they screw up will become afraid of doing irreparable damage to others.

My childhood fears about growing up had been realized: I could see the evil in me, I could see the damage I could cause in other people's lives by not resisting evil. There was a concern at one point in my life that I would one day make a mistake so big, intentionally or not, that many people would be irreparably damaged by my actions. This led me to conclude, for a brief moment, that the world would be better without me.

I had to step aside and look at my place in the world, the part I've played so far, and the effects of my presence. I was reminded of everyone who said they've been blessed by having me around. I came to realize that God knows what each of us are capable of, and it was His decision to allow us into this world, even knowing that we would often choose evil over good.

The fear of screwing things up is probably most common in people who recognize their potential—leaders, artists, warriors, speakers. We recognize the good we can do and the damage we can cause if we don't resist evil, and on top of that we know our weaknesses.

I look at myself and the people in whom I see potential, and I draw this conclusion: the damage we can cause by trying and screwing up is not as great as the good that will never be if we do nothing at all.

This belief encourages me to keep trying.

A MATTER OF HONOUR

For a long time, I've been afraid to make any sort of promise to God. I have a general fear of making promises, even ones I'm pretty sure I can keep, simply because I never know what will happen. Events are always out of my control. And I know what it feels like to be promised something only to have the person go back on their word.

I've had the same reasoning about my service to God—I will do the best I can, to the best of my ability, but I won't make any promises. I won't swear to always do what I'm asked, only what I *can* do. (As if God would ask me to do more than I'm capable of doing.)

I have told God that I would follow Him all my days, but I refused to make my servitude a promise, in case something ever happened and I inadvertently broke that promise. I have to ask myself: whose honour am I really concerned about by not making promises to God? Is it for His honour, or mine?

There's a difference between serving your master as sacrificially as possible to gain honour through it, and serving your master as sacrificially as possible for the honour of your master and your master alone, with no regard to your own name.

The ultimate truth is that my name and my identity aren't my own. Everything I am is a gift from God; He can take it all away should He choose to. Why do I act as though my reputation is something I've earned? As though my name is my responsibility alone? Has not God provided both the abilities and opportunities to gain what reputation I have? Do I not owe Him everything, including my name?

Do I really position God's honour above my own? Am I willing to put my honour on the line for the sake of His? Would I willingly suffer dishonour in order to bring honour to Him?

I fear that if I make a promise to serve Him and then break it, my honour will be stained. But if I fully surrender all that I am to God, I acknowledge that everything I am, including my name and my honour, belongs to God. I also acknowledge that I'm not in control—God is. Would He then deliberately put me in a position where I have no choice but to break my promise to serve Him? As long as I fight for control of my life, and my honour, I'm trying to sail against the wind. When I acknowledge that all I am is His, and surrender it all to Him, I will finally be used for the purposes He ultimately created me for.

My honour is not my own—my honour is in God's hands, to break or mend as He sees fit. Surrendered to Him, He will use it in whatever way will bring Him the most glory and honour. If His honour is my greatest priority, this is the only route to take.

It's time to stop being proud, to stop saying, "I'm not good enough; therefore I promise nothing." God has not asked me to be anything more than what I am. So I now give Him all of what I am. What I *can be* is now in His hands.

CHAPTER EIGHT
Sociality

I am the son, and the heir,
Of a shyness that is criminally vulgar.
—The Smiths, *How Soon Is Now?*

A social life is recognized as one of the most difficult things for an autistic to establish—even high-functioning autistics.

A common problem is that we don't recognize the facial cues telling us what a person is feeling. The different combinations of raised or frowning eyebrows and grins or open-lip smiles make little sense to us. We cannot interpret the meaning of different vocal tones, either, or word choices that to most people would signify hidden messages.

I still struggle with all of the above, though I've come much further in understanding emotional responses than most autistics. Oddly, I'm able to interpret responses on movies and TV shows just as well as anybody. That may be because those are actors directed to give certain responses, which they do very well. In real life, people aren't as revealing of their emotions, and it becomes much harder to interpret them. When watching unscripted TV shows, I'm still in the dark.

I struggle to attach a particular name to a particular face and particular actions. In other words, I might bump into someone and recognize their face but not remember their name or why they're important. Or I might recognize a name but not remember what the person looks like or what they've done. Many people have had the experience of walking up to me expecting familiarity and finding that I treat them like an unknown.

I've wondered if I have a low opinion of others. I've noticed that most people seem unimportant to me. I don't know if that's normal, or normal for people of the TV generation, but I see similarities between how I watch TV and the way I view people around me.

The majority of people I see when I go out are just "extras"; they have no specific role, they're just fillers. If someone has a "speaking role," then I'm supposed to pay attention to what they say since it may be significant for me. But I have to really get to know a person's story before I consider them relevant. Once I know a person well enough, I recognize their importance whether I like the person or not or think they're boring.

Ideally, one would recognize God's hand in the lives of all the people one meets, recognize that God cares as much about these people as He does anyone. This is stuff I know if I think about it logically, but it hasn't become a natural, heartfelt instinct yet.

COMMUNICATION

I have certain standards when it comes to socializing, which nobody else ever follows. And yet I continue to hold to that standard because it is perfectly logical to me. It's as if I grew up in another culture, still adhering to those rules and expecting the same of others. This may be a remnant of my centre-of-the-universe mentality.

One example is that I don't expect people to respond to every email I send out, since many of my emails are just thoughts that I want to share. But when I ask someone a specific question, I expect to be answered. I don't mind if it takes a few days to get back to me, but when the person does email me, ignoring the question I asked, I'm offended.

By now I've concluded that people in the real world expect me to drop a subject when they don't reply to it. But since conversation pieces are often forgotten in the busyness of daily life, I can't assume that a question has been ignored, which means I have to ask it again. If a person is simply unwilling or unable to answer the question, I have no objection to them saying so. I myself have had to tell people, "I want to change the subject," because I know discussing that subject will conjure up resentful feelings in me. When I ask a question, I can accept someone replying with, "I won't answer that." What offends me is when they pretend the question was never asked.

I think the rule others follow is to simply ignore it and change the subject, because saying "I won't answer that" arouses suspicion. But since I catch when a question is ignored, it arouses suspicion anyway—and insults my intelligence.

I'm more graceful these days. I don't get super-ticked at people who don't answer every question I send them. But be aware that many high-functioning autistics might.

Certain topics make me angry to talk about. Even when people are just trying to help, I find that feelings of resentment rise up in me for people who insist on talking about them. I'm not justifying my resentment. I know it's wrong; I'm simply acknowledging that this is what happens when people tread past the barriers I mark out for them. It would be wrong, and hazardous to friendships, for me to ignore the feelings that arise when people dwell on those topics, so I warn them; I don't want glitches between us.

I hold nothing against the people who cross these lines without knowing a line has been drawn. But when people persist on a topic I've told them to step away from, I have a right to be angry.

MESSAGES

I've noted that typing, in books and in emails, is an important form of communication for me. I wouldn't say it's my favourite, since face-to-face conversations are far more personal, but there are aspects of typed communication that I cannot get in any other form.

I've seen counsellors hold up cardboard imitations of keyboards for autistics to spell out their thoughts, so I know there's a common thread in here somewhere. I'm not sure why most autistics communicate so well with a keyboard and cannot speak with their mouths. I find that sometimes what I need to say is just too detailed, too exact to be spoken in the moment. I need the time to think about what I want to say, and then make sure I have it right. Under the pressure of live chatter, I cannot get my words together quite the way they need to be received.

Perhaps for most autistics the use of a keyboard (digital or imitation) creates an indirect, and therefore comfortable, means of sending a message.

DISCOMFORT WITH PEOPLE

In my childhood, I believed that people choose what they look like. (This was not a problem for me since I looked exactly how I wanted to.) If someone was ugly, it was because they wanted to be ugly; if someone was scary, it was because they were mean and wanted to scare me; if someone was old, it was because they wanted to be old. The same went for being a girl or being a different race.

I remember physically attacking one kid because he looked like a jerk. I remember once assaulting him when he had his posse with him. That didn't scare me; I was gonna take on all his thugs. In hindsight they seemed rather peaceable.

I remember seeing a deformed person in a wheelchair struggling to get into a store. My mother held the door open for them, and I asked my mom why, since to look the way they did they were obviously a nasty person. I also remember not liking black people. My sister Anna confronted me about this and said that she had a black friend who was a very nice person. That made no sense to me. It took a while for it to really sink in, but that was the beginning of my realization that people's control over their appearance is limited—and that my race wasn't the only good one. It was longer still before I realized that many people of different races are actually quite good-looking!

It seems that without the right upbringing, I would have grown to be a massive bigot.

I'm ashamed to say that I don't handle people of difference well. Even fellow autistics can make me uncomfortable. Maybe it's just a psychological aspect of being reminded, in a very vivid way, of where I come from. It's not something I do intentionally, but nor do I know how to stop thinking this way. Race is visually obvious to me. If a person has darker skin than me, I can't help but notice.

Now, judging someone based on their race is short-sighted, but is the act of acknowledging their race a bad thing in itself? Shouldn't differences be affirmed as points of pride for all people involved?

For some reason, I still feel discomfort around people of certain races. I hope that won't be the case after I've seen more of the world. It's possible that my discomfort with other races is partly due to not spending enough time with a wide variety of people.

SMILING

It's next to impossible for me to multitask. I can focus on only one thing at a time. Even when required to do multiple things at once, I can only do that by starting one thing, then the other, and only if the first thing, once started, requires no supervision.

The issue is focus. I have a very strong focus, but it can only be tuned to one thing at a time.

That's another reason why I socialize much better one-on-one than in a group. With a single person, I can observe and respond to subtle cues like tone, eye contact, body language, and diction—because they're all coming from one source. In a group setting, there are several sources of tone, diction, and body language, so I don't know where to focus. I can hear everything that's going on, and I know each word everyone says, but I'm unable to make anything out of it... other than the blatant. I don't pick up on hidden messages, words within words, or how each person reacts to every word.

Another challenge is that my face responds to things much slower than my brain does. In a situation where most people would smile out of politeness, my face remains neutral. My face doesn't smile in response to another person. This isn't because I fail to acknowledge that they're smiling, but because my face doesn't smile unless I tell it to, and I don't tell myself to smile until I've processed that I need to smile, and by that time the occasion to smile is usually passed.

In the rare event that an occasion to smile lasts long enough for me to process it, I'm capable of forcing a smile. However, this often feels contrived, and I try to avoid making contrived smiles.

LISTENING

I'm capable of paying considerable attention to a person when they speak, but this doesn't happen all the time. Having A.D.D. doesn't mean I'm incapable of focusing; it just means my point of focus tends to change repeatedly. In my worst moments, I'll ask someone a question and immediately start thinking about something else so I don't even hear the answer. I'll ask someone, "What time do you want to meet?" and immediately think, "What should my Charizard's fourth move be?"

HUMOUR

It's been debated whether or not I have a sense of humour. Sometimes a person will say something in jest but do it with a straight face because their sense of humour is "dry." Unless I'm able to read between the lines, I won't know they're joking. Sometimes I *can* tell they're joking, straight-faced or otherwise, but I respond to them seriously anyway, making them think I didn't get it. This is because as a child my face never showed emotion and my voice was always (and still is) monotone, which made the ridiculous things I said all the funnier to people who responded best to "dry humour."

As a child who enjoyed laughter, the only universal language I understood, I learned to respond to everything with the same dry expression. The problem is I do it so well that people often mistake me for being serious when I'm actually kidding. The result is that many of the jokes I tell to someone unfamiliar with me are lost to the wind. My father and I have had this unfortunate problem for some time. We're both quite funny, if only we knew it!

Stand-up comedy, for example, is all about looking at what we call "normal" and pointing out how ridiculous and illogical "normal" really is. This is done most effectively with a neutral voice—you don't have to sound goofy, because people get it—normal *is* the joke. In fact, the more neutral your voice, the funnier it is, because you sound like someone who's genuinely trying to understand why the world works the way it does.

I've observed that, other than diction, church sermons and stand-up comedy have a lot in common.

The most memorable stand-up routines involve talking to the crowd about what's wrong with the world—you know, the stuff we all think is normal and okay because we've been taught to think that. When the comic just describes a product, or job, or social rule, or law, you come to realize how stupid it is. They don't even have to exaggerate. All they have to do is talk about it exactly as it is and suddenly your eyes are opened. "Yeah! That *is* stupid! How come it took so long for me to see that?"

There's a story about someone from a popular magazine who got into hot water with a certain religious leader, not for insulting him or his faith but simply for repeating something the religious leader had said—because that was all the information you needed to know what was wrong with his teachings. The most effective way to point out how stupid someone is, is to quote them.

I've frequently been reprimanded for my ridiculously bad timing. The problem is that once I get comfortable with someone, I'm just too funny. Actually, when it comes to humour, my sense of timing is well-practiced. I'm very good at delivering a punchline at the time it will be funniest. The problem is that I haven't yet learned to keep my mouth shut when someone is eating or drinking.

A new problem is that I'll be talking nonchalantly, secretly setting up a joke, and then just as I'm about to deliver the punchline the person I'm talking to will take a big sip of their drink, and I'll freeze and wait for them to swallow. My friends know what this means, then laugh and choke on their drink anyway. I don't see a way around it.

RELATIONSHIPS

Relationships among autistics are very few. First, there is the social barrier itself, the difficulty in making any kind of connection. Then there's the issue of maintaining the connection. I know a lot of people, but I only consider a few to be friends. I consider everybody else an acquaintance.

Here's how I define the difference between a friend and an acquaintance. I consider someone a friend if we know things about each other that an acquaintance would not know. This doesn't necessarily mean deep, dark secrets—it means we care enough about each other to want to know the "boring" stuff. An acquaintance asks how you're doing and expects a certain cliché answer. A friend asks how you're doing and expects an honest, in-depth answer. This may or may not have started as a defence mechanism. Either way, the idea is to separate the people who care about me from the people who only want to look like they care.

For years, I've tried to get to the point where I could consider myself a friend to a certain girl (in her eyes we were possibly already friends, but not in my eyes). Whenever I asked how she was doing or if she needed prayer for anything, her response was always, "Everything's perfect." No matter how many times I tried to get to know her, I couldn't consider myself anything more than an acquaintance if I didn't know anything about her beyond what she looked and sounded like—everybody knew those things.

The day came when I unintentionally upset her. I gave her some advice on how her art could be made better. It seemed harmless enough, and complimentary, but I didn't realize how deeply personal her art was. I was able to talk to her about it afterward and patch things up.

I don't know how else to say this, but I'm glad it happened. I'm not glad that it upset her, but I'm glad that I finally knew something about her. I finally knew what she cared about; I understood how she looked at her art. I could finally consider myself her friend.

In my youth group days, I would never walk into a group of peers and expect to be welcomed—even if I knew people in the group. It felt too much like an intrusion. I didn't think people wanted me around. I'm trying to put myself forward more often now. Usually I won't unless there are at least two friends in the group. I'm trying to get it into my head that my friends like me and like having me around.

People with autism struggle to socialize with their own age group. This is much more apparent in childhood than in adult years, only because the age difference is more apparent when you're a kid.

Although I find it much more meaningful to focus on one individual at a time than to have to think about the social needs of an entire group, that much focus may be what scares some people away.

Despite not socializing well myself, I have an uncanny understanding of how human interaction works. I think being on the outside, so to speak, of the social world allows me to study it objectively. When someone has a crush, I know the difference between love and admiration.

I have never been in a romantic relationship, but people in relationships have told me that my understanding of relationships has helped them understand their own. Of course, my insight is obviously limited to what I'm able to observe. And personal experience is not always the best position for observation.

I'm fascinated with power, understanding how one obtains power, and how power transfers from one person to another. I've seen it happen several times in groups, solely through the process of social interaction. I've felt myself gain power, and felt it taken from me very tangibly.

At one point, a friendship of mine was falling apart because I had sent this person multiple emails and received no reply. I was hurt because I'd once had a good friendship with this person, and it appeared as though they didn't care to keep it going. I wanted to keep attempting to contact them, but the silence already hurt me so much. I thought to myself, *I've done my part. It's up to them now to show an effort to keep this friendship going.*

And then I thought, *But what if they don't? What if they really are too lazy or too stupid to put in that effort? Will I really let this relationship go just because "I've done my part?" If this person is being a complete idiot and doesn't realize what they're letting slip away, is the fact that I've already made a contribution justification for me to now sit back and let this happen?*

I sent one final message, reminding the person of the friendship we had, letting them know I wanted to keep that, letting them know how their silence made me feel, but informing them that I could not put up with this cold shoulder any longer. Fortunately, I got a response that brought the friendship back together. I've had to send that kind of message out more than once, though, and the results aren't always positive.

Honesty

One notable trait of mine is honesty. I don't always pick up on hints when someone is trying to say something without saying it. I don't do well at mind games, which may be why women tend to get annoyed with me, and not just women my age. I need people to tell me directly what they want or need, instead of expecting me to have it figured out.

I don't know if it's my lack of observing my surroundings or just a lack of empathy, but I rarely know what someone else needs unless they tell me directly.

I ran into this a lot with my sisters. One of them would suddenly burst out with, "*I'll* do the dishes." Then I would ask if they wanted help, and they would say, with a sigh, "No, it's fine." Of course, now that I'm older, I know what that means. But the reason I couldn't help them when they said they didn't want help was that I still struggled with the fear of getting in the way. I feared acting independently unless directly asked for assistance.

That brought on a lot of guilt, which hurt because I genuinely didn't know how to change, and still don't. I need to be told where the need is before I move into action. I made the decision that if no one was willing to ask for help, then there was no reason to feel guilty.

Now I have more of a humorous approach. When I've been standing around doing nothing and somebody says "Thanks for helping," I say, "You're welcome." Even when I know something is going on and people need assistance, I still can't figure out from observation what's needed. I have to walk up to the person in charge and say, "I'm here to do whatever you need—just let me know."

All that said, I know I'm not the only one who suffers when people fail to communicate properly. I've seen too many relationships fall apart because of bad communication. People constantly assume that the other person can read their mind. I don't know where this idea comes from, but everybody seems to believe it. People say one thing but mean something else, or they assume they shouldn't have to say anything at all. Everyone has forgotten what they learned in kindergarten—"Use your words!"

This is particularly recurrent in romantic relationships. When someone meets the person of their dreams and falls madly in love, they come to believe that they're so meant for each other that talking is unnecessary. Can you see what happens next?

"I shouldn't have to say what I feel; they should know automatically. That's what soul mates do."

Even if you were meant for each other, to assume that communication is unnecessary is unrealistic. The kind of relationship where you know each other inside-out takes time. It takes years to observe all possible nuances. It's unreasonable to assume that full knowledge will occur instantly.

When the other person asks what's wrong, it's because they genuinely don't know and want to learn. Asking what the problem is demonstrates a willingness to learn what upsets the other person and what makes them happy. To hurt them with the silent treatment because they "ought to know without asking" is to put them on a pedestal far too lofty. They're the one fighting to keep the relationship alive. This appears to be a global pandemic.

Another issue I have with people being indirect with each other is that it creates an environment of pretence and an excuse for superficiality, an environment in which we don't have to say what we mean or mean what we say, an environment in which nobody can admit mistakes, problems, or struggles.

I can't stand pretence. Too many people are afraid to tell me the real reason they won't talk. They'd much rather act as if nothing is wrong when in reality their lives are falling apart. I can't help anyone who won't tell me what the problem is—and I can't ignore when someone's hurting and won't ask for help.

When people ask me how I'm doing, I tell them. "I'm tired." "I have a headache." "I'm nervous." "I'm alright." "I'm not that good." "I'm not sure."

Sometimes I really don't know how I'm doing. Either I've been too focused on something else to pay attention to how I'm feeling or I've experienced too many ups and downs in a short amount of time for me to accurately say. Sometimes I answer with a quick "Okay" because the question is addressed to me as the person is walking away. I get the feeling they don't care enough to hear what I'm saying anyway.

I have been told by a Christian friend that everyone walks around with a veil over their faces—a mask, a façade. And I'm the only person she knows who doesn't wear a veil.

This goes back to something I read in *Wild at Heart*, that everyone has an alter ego, a mask they wear to avoid people seeing who they really are. Sometimes we assume this alternate persona so well that we convince ourselves that we're someone else. This can last until we're finally exposed for who we really are. If you're less fortunate, you could go your whole life without anyone finding out, living your whole life as someone else.

When wearing the mask we never allow ourselves to be who God made us to be. We insist on being someone else. Or we refuse to admit imperfection, even though Jesus called the unrighteous, not the righteous, to redemption. The truth is that God can make us into who He has intended us to be, but first we have to admit who we are not.

When reading that section of *Wild at Heart*, I genuinely couldn't think of a mask I was wearing, even after asking my friends and family. I know why now. It's because I had already made the decision growing up to make honesty one of my top priorities, and that has never changed. If anything, I've struggled with the persona others want to attach to me. It's frustrating to be an open, honest person in this world, because everybody works with the assumption that you are not who you say you are.

Too often I've asked a question the person wouldn't answer, only because they assumed I was asking for a hidden reason. Sometimes a question is just a question, but people become evasive or defensive, thinking I have some ulterior motive for asking. No matter how hard I try to get through to people that I am what they see, that I wear no masks, that I have no ulterior motive, most people never get it.

One time, as my family was preparing for a road trip, I asked my mother, "Do you have bandaids in your purse?"

Her response was, "Aren't there any in the bathroom?"

That didn't answer my question, but her response left me to assume that she would only ask her question if she had no bandaids in her purse.

So I checked the bathroom drawer. There were some large bandaids, but nothing suitable for traveling.

When I saw her again (still in the house), she asked if I had found any bandaids in the bathroom.

"Yes," I said. "But I want to know if we have any we can take with us."

To which she replied, "Ah. That's not what you asked, is it?"

I believe my exact words were "Do you have bandaids in your purse?" If I had wanted to know if there were any bandaids anywhere, I would have asked, "Are there any bandaids anywhere in the world?"

As you've probably guessed, she did in fact have bandaids in her purse, and she was aware of it, which should have made my question very easy to answer. Had she just answered the question I asked instead of answering a different question entirely, we both could have saved a lot of time.

Of course, I didn't start a debate with her about it; women have a way of making me wrong when I'm not.

My sisters and I often run into situations where they're upset because of something I said. I try to calm them down, but nothing I say gets through. The slightest ill choice of words can lead to a massive misunderstanding where they think they've offended me and I think I've offended them and we each feel guilty for what we've done while at the same time feel like the other is wrong for feeling the way they feel.

Sometimes I see what's going on and try to stop it. I try to say, "It's all right" or "It's not that bad" or "Nobody did anything wrong," but in the emotional tornado words are often unheeded.

In situations like that, all I can do is hug them, or give them a kiss, or hold their hand—something to show continuing affection despite whatever we're struggling with. When we find ourselves in a place where words are useless, physical actions are the only form of communication we understand. It's my way of saying, "I still love you. No matter what's happened, or what you think I said, know this—I love you."

Karen and I had both a lot of love and a lot of friction growing up. In the years shortly before she moved out and got married, there was a lot more friction and a lot less grace. In the first few years of her marriage, I felt as though an impenetrable wall had been built up between us. I didn't like it.

One day, I sat her down and had a heart-to-heart talk with her. I addressed many of the issues we'd had in the past, and explained that I didn't feel that way anymore, that I was sorry for anything I had done to hurt her.

She was surprised, to say the least, but she was used to me being different. After that, our relationship improved. We understood each other much more clearly. All bitterness was done away with. I got back the sister I used to laugh and play with.

Not everyone can handle honesty at that deep a level, to actually address problems that have been ignored and covered with pretence. If you can manage to walk through that with someone, in grace, acknowledging the issues and realizing that they need not be a cause for separation, I think you'll find that those relationships can weather anything.

I have a theory that the relationships most likely to last are the ones where both individuals see the worst in each other early on, and get through it. The longer a relationship continues under the assumption that either individual is perfect, the more disastrous it will be when the first problem comes along.

SUFFERING

There is one occasion when I was experiencing an urgent, desperate, and painful spiritual conflict. After a lingering lack of communication and a series of severe misunderstandings and emotional eruptions, it looked like a split in the family was a real danger. A dividing line had been drawn where no real barrier existed, but people in the family were already taking sides. Despite my best efforts to open communications and bring clarity to some strong misunderstandings, it looked like one more shove was all my family needed to fall beyond the point of repair. And it was being demanded of me that I choose a side, though I was trying very hard not to.

All I could do was email my church prayer team, without giving specific details. I then spent a whole day in desperate prayer for God's intervention.

After a day, everyone's emotions calmed considerably. Communications were opened up again and they were done with grace. Misunderstandings were clarified and mended, to my exhausted relief. That period of turmoil was the darkest my soul has ever felt.

Clearly this was evident in my email to the church, since I had written and sent it while in the middle of the crisis. Surprisingly, though, I received no replies to the email. I sent out a second email to let everyone know that all was well, but also (somewhat emotionally) to express confusion over the lack of responses. Some people responded then—rather defensively—which surprised me more.

I've put the hurt behind me, but it raised an interesting insight which I've carried since then. This wasn't the first time someone had been offended by something I said while in emotional anguish, and I find that rather short-sighted. I'm not saying I wasn't rude by making the comment; I'm just saying that when you're in that much pain—and in some cases it's taking all your energy just to hold on to sanity, resist suicide, resist turning your back on God—you shouldn't be expected to waste energy on manners.

Now that I have experience, both with my own trial and even helping others get through times of severe spiritual and emotional anguish, I understand better what happens to the soul during those dark periods. And I know that being polite is the last thing on your mind.

Yes, when someone neglects their manners, they are likely to be more open about what they really think. Even still, I try not to take it as the full truth, especially if they're only expressing their angry thoughts at the time. Although their soul is torn wide open for all to see, it's also not in one piece. They may be so overcome by blind rage or despair that they don't see any light from anyone.

I've since adopted the policy that when someone is in that state, they're exempt from the expectation of being polite. I hope others will offer me the same grace. In order to stay away from the blame and guilt mentality, I pretty much have to give myself permission to forget manners when I'm in that state.

LONELINESS

I've never had a girlfriend.

I may not be as social as most people, but I still have the need for a romantic relationship. My current state of singleness is not a choice. I just haven't found a woman who gets me. And that's what I'm looking for—a deep connection. A one night stand won't do it for me; I'll feel worse if she doesn't stay.

I don't even really know what I'm looking for in a woman, except that I haven't found it yet. I used to have a fairly extensive list of attractive traits, but what I care about most today is simply finding a woman who's willing to communicate with me. I've had good friendships fall apart just because the other person suddenly wasn't interesting in communicating anymore.

Also, getting my sense of humour is probably a must, otherwise I foresee a lot of awkward silences.

I always try to get to know people as friends first, before getting into anything more intimate. This is harder than it should be in most cases.

One problem I've had in the past is being too forward with women; my logical side works very slowly whereas my creative side works faster, thinking of all possible outcomes of a conversation. I've gotten to thinking romantically before I really knew the person.

These days, I try hard to keep a lid on my romantic side. I still seem to scare women off, however, and it may be that I focus on them too strongly as we talk. That's why I've decided that the best scenario for getting to know women is to be around more than one at a time; that way, my focus can shift between one and the other. The number of men makes no difference. They're not as important.

I've come to notice that most women I become acquainted with fill me with a sense of obligation, and I think they detect that. The sense of obligation is always counterproductive. If a woman is single, I must woo her, but I'm naturally shy when it comes to women. Yet I feel as though I must push past that in order to do the manly thing and show at least partial interest even if the interest isn't that strong.

I have since realized that any time that sense of obligation comes up, it's a good sign that this woman isn't right for me, which theoretically should allow me to calm down and be myself again. When the right one comes along, affectionate behaviour will be natural, not an obligation. I won't be able to help myself, as opposed to forcing myself.

It's not about sex anymore; it's just about having someone there. It's about having a partner for life, someone I can confer with as I deal with my struggles. A second opinion from someone I trust, who knows me and my needs as well as I know myself.

The need for sex is general, but I'm not the kind of person to just have casual sex. Considering what's involved in the act, I couldn't do something that exposing with anyone I wasn't completely comfortable with.

CHAPTER NINE
My Discoveries

I know well what lies beyond my sleeping refuge,
The nightmare I built my own world to escape.
—Evanescence, *Imaginary*

ON AUTISM

I once saw a documentary in which a mother had twin daughters. One was autistic, the other was not. One performed at the average level as a child, but the other would sit in front of the computer all day, licking her fingers and touching the computer screen as if finger-painting.

What really upset me was the attitude of the mother in the way she compared the two children, saying, "This one is functioning properly. She's contributing. She's being productive. The other one just wastes her day at the computer."

I know it's difficult for parents to accept that their child is autistic; it's a perfectly natural and God-honouring thing to want the best for your child. What upsets me is that this mother seemed to appraise one child over the other based on productivity. She didn't bother to *try* understanding her own daughter.

Have you ever observed how a small amount of liquid affects a computer screen? Or a television screen? It bends the light being emitted from the screen, resulting in different colours and images.

It was blatantly obvious to me why this girl did what she did. She was manipulating the screen to create her own art form. That's cognitive thinking, not random movements. Whether anybody else could see her art or not, this girl was an artist.

After observing my own life and experiences, and observing the behaviour of other autistics, I've concluded that our behaviours are choices. There are chemical and biological factors, of course, accounting for the particular way our brains are wired, but things like echolalia, self-abuse, and withdrawal all have the appearance of being conscious decisions, even if we don't know why we make them, even if it's gotten to the point that we can't consciously control our bodies—all of these activities appear to be responses to something.

We're already very different from the crowd. We can't control things like the speed at which we process the world, or how we process the world, but there is evidence of autistics learning to control behavioural factors.

I can testify that even after getting to the point where I was aware of the real world, I was aware that I was different from other kids. Most autistics may not know how to articulate it, but when we are aware of other people we are also aware that we are inadequate. Withdrawal and similar behaviours are automatic responses to this. Either that, or we find that existence is simply easier when we don't have to deal with reality.

I'm not suggesting that autism is nothing more than extreme escapism— there are definite physical differences between us and everyone else—but retreating into one's own world is much easier as an autistic, and sometimes, aware that we are different, we see no reason to be in the real world even when we have the choice.

From my own memories, and from observing videos of other autistics, I see that we will intentionally separate from a group, hide in a corner, or leave the room, content just being with ourselves. We'll even withdraw emotionally if necessary, cutting off our connection to someone when it becomes uncomfortable.

Severe autistics may be trapped in their own world, trying to get out but not knowing the way, but I think higher-functioning autistics have enough awareness of our environment to be able to make the choice.

Studying *Nobody Nowhere*, by Donna Williams, gives further evidence of this. In her own words, Donna as a child viewed "the world" as separate from her, nonsensical, and oftentimes terrifying and hostile. She was fully content being in her own world, getting lost in lights and colours, and hated when anything from the "real world" interfered— such as hunger. Echolalia was her attempt at communicating with "the world." Whatever words were spoken to her, though she didn't understand them, she interpreted as attempts to communicate, so by repeating them she believed she showed her own effort to communicate. This response, however, was often met by a slap, as her mother had no understanding of autistic behaviour.

Frustration with "the world's" intolerance of her led Donna to find far greater peace in her own world for many years.

For me, I struggle with the fear of responsibility, which I want to overcome. I know I'll have to before I can do much of what I hope to do with my life. It again comes back to my failure to sort out what the world expects of me, what I expect of myself, and what God expects of me. Only one of those matters.

I don't consider myself better than most autistics. Not all of my decisions have been for the best, either. Dealing with pressure and anxiety, the feeling of inadequacy, the temptation to withdraw, and the fear of regression are all ongoing battles for me. Many of my decisions have been for my progress, but I still struggle with making right decisions.

I don't know if this has anything to do with autism, but I respond very negatively to being pushed. Severe autistics aren't pushed onward; people don't expect anything of them more than what they are. People didn't expect much from me, and so didn't push me to be anything more. But now I have people pushing me this way and that, thinking I'm not living up to my potential, and because of my struggles with pressure and anxiety, I take it very negatively.

Severe autistics push themselves onward. I pushed myself onward as a child, because nobody else did. Left alone, it would be a lot easier to make the right decisions for the right reasons, and have peace that they're the right decisions. But with everybody hounding me to be something more than what I feel equipped to be, I feel crushed by the pressure.

WOLF PEOPLE

One day, I discovered what I call "wolf people," people who are able to "sniff out" lameness. They meet someone and quickly determine whether or not that person is cool. If that person is cool, they like them; if not, they don't. It's that simple. Once a wolf person has made their decision as to whether you're lame or cool, it's near impossible to get them to change their mind about you. First impressions are everything to a wolf person.

You can learn to spot them. They're typically the people who are most uncomfortable when the person next to them is doing something incredibly lame, like telling a lame joke. Depending on how much grace the wolf person has, they may manage an awkward laugh or glare murderously at the offender.

A lot of teenagers are wolf people, very few grownups are, and even fewer little kids. I think the ability to sniff out lameness is a defence against disappointment. If a person feels they've been betrayed or let down too often, they'll learn to detect falsehood and separate themselves from it. People who are considered cool are also (usually) considered to be honest, though not honest by legalistic standards such as never telling a lie; they're honest by the standard of being true to themselves and kindred spirits. By the time you're a teenager, the dominant belief is that everyone is a jerk, so the only people who are trustworthy are the ones with the honesty to admit that they're jerks, which often makes one "cool." Thus the theory goes (if you're a wolf person) that if somebody is cool, they can also be trusted, which is not as true as it should be.

The exact age at which a child develops the sense varies between individual personalities and experiences, but it surfaces most often in the teen years. Few kids have been disappointed enough times for it to sink in that they need to learn for themselves who they can trust. But by their teen years, most have had too many disappointments in life.

By adulthood, most people become dissatisfied with the wolf lifestyle, having failed to find a kindred spirit who could be trusted. (The jerk who admitted to being a jerk turned out to be a jerk.) So we give in to the fateful belief that everyone is fake, that the world functions on fake people, and that in order to be a part of it we have to be fake, too. By this time, living as a wolf person is considered unrealistic and irresponsible; it's an attempt at escapism from the reality of a world where nobody can be trusted. Adults learn to numb their lameness detector in order to function in the world.

That, from my observations, is the connection between coolness and honesty, but there's also the connection between lameness and falsehood. Consider that one of the lamest things a person can do is pretend to be funny. If a person is pretending to be funny, they're putting on a façade of being socially gifted because they don't want people to perceive them as being socially inadequate. I think all forms of lameness are the result of trying to hide, trying to be something you're not. Therefore, it sets off alarms for anyone trying to detect falsehood.

I used to be uncomfortable around infants, and I know I'm not alone in this. When a person is a newborn, there is a sense that they are "fresh from God" and have not yet seen what evil the world is capable of. I was afraid of them seeing this evil in me, because babies are more capable than anyone of detecting lameness, having recently come from God's presence and not yet been seriously corrupted by the world. Infants have an awareness of things adults can't typically sense.

Children have this awareness for several months at least. I'm guessing it gradually dissipates and gives way to the naivety of little kids, before the terrible twos.

Teenagers, having been constantly disappointed, desperately want this awareness back but don't know how to return to the innocence of early childhood, so they develop their own detection system and become wolf people.

By the time you're an adult, the wolf person lifestyle is usually found to be inefficient in achieving what was hoped, as there are just too many fake people in the world and even fellow wolf people are too corrupted to change that. So this awareness is something that babies are born with, kids gradually lose, teenagers try to get back, and adults give up on ever finding.

Should you find yourself in the company of wolf people, and you know you're emitting lameness, the best thing to do is admit that lameness and take on a submissive attitude.

This is taken right from the animal kingdom. When one wolf challenges another wolf and realizes the other is stronger, he lowers his head, baring his neck (the killing spot) to the other wolf. Usually the other wolf will give a signal allowing the submissive one to rise and no blood is shed.

Good wolf people will respect even a lame person, if that lame person admits to their own lameness. Make sure you do this honestly, though, without overdoing it, or you'll just offend them more.

I have found myself in positions of lameness many times, usually from having to do something I suck at, and I know the wolf people can sniff me out. Admitting lameness usually works.

I used to see myself as a wolf person, but I don't think that would be accurate of me now. Although I still have that sense of smell, I usually have enough grace to give people multiple chances to be cool. Many pastors and elders I've met in church have set off my lameness alarms when I first met them. Let's face it: most people in leadership positions within a church are expected to be something they're not—sinless. But I gave these guys a chance and later learned that they had very real spiritual gifts that could only have come from God. These guys knew exactly what I needed to hear when I needed to hear it.

God has taught me that even though a person may be lame by my standards, some are still dedicated to God. God can still use them for His purposes.

MODESTY

I've come to realize that modesty is wrong. Modesty, as I've seen it used, amounts to downplaying one's own worth in front of others for the sake of not appearing big-headed. People are modest when they know they're awesome, and they know that everyone else knows they're awesome, but they're afraid of people disliking them because of their pride. So they downplay their worth to eliminate any reason for someone disliking them.

Modesty is also a sign that someone still views themselves as their own creation. If everyone is a creation of God, then downplaying the worth of anyone, including yourself, is wrong. God wants your awesomeness to shine because you reflect the awesomeness of your Creator.

The ideal solution is to accept your awesomeness, not pretend it isn't there, and at the same time acknowledge the awesomeness of others. Instead of downplaying yourself and saying, "No, I'm really just as crappy as you are," recognize the giftedness that both of you have and say, "We're both awesome! How awesome is the God who made us!"

Humility, on the other hand, is good.

Humility, though not arrogant, has nothing to do with downplaying one's self worth. You don't have to view yourself as crappy to be humble. Humility amounts to having an accurate perception of oneself in relation to an Almighty God. In humility you can still recognize your awesomeness for what it is; you're simply aware that it is infinitesimal next to God's. Humility in social interactions is being respectful of others and their awesomeness, because we are all made in God's image. But it doesn't mean letting people walk all over you, because you bear God's image as well.

Humility is carrying out one of Jesus's commands to us, which is to treat everyone as we would treat Him.

I don't write this to put anyone down. Modesty is something we as Canadians have been trained to embrace—and at first glance it seems perfectly fine. Many times in my life I fear I've been more modest and less humble, because I still viewed myself as my own creation and not God's creation—one of many causes of my perfectionism. This is something I want to reverse in my life. This is me analyzing the reasons behind what we do, and looking for a better solution.

LIKE A ROBOT

Of all the characters in fiction, the one I associate with best is Data, an android, from *Star Trek: The Next Generation*. Since I've started watching that show again, I've noticed just how similar his behaviour is to mine. Data does not get humans; he doesn't understand their emotions or the nuances of their speech. If someone is sarcastic with him, he doesn't know it. If someone is being silly, he doesn't get it. If someone is having a problem, he doesn't perceive it. This is the way I am in most situations.

The crew of the *Enterprise*, the ship Data is posted to, has learned Data's behaviour. They've learned how to interact with him. Surprisingly, even people who have known me my whole life haven't learned how to interact with me.

While speaking with the doctor, Data once casually mentioned his exceptional skills at a certain task, simply stating fact. The doctor seemed put off. Later Data turned to Commander Riker, who had witnessed the interaction, and asked, "Did the doctor think I was bragging?"

Most people would reply, "Oh no. I'm sure she's fine. She knows you didn't mean anything by it." Riker, on the other hand, said something like, "Yeah, probably."

Most people would patronize, but then Data would learn nothing. Riker knew Data well enough to understand what he needed to hear, so Data would know better in the future.

People don't realize that when I do things that upset others, I genuinely don't *know* that it bothers anyone. People generally conclude that if I'm really that rude, there's no point telling me it's wrong, or if I'm really that stupid, there's no point trying to explain it. They think the best thing is to say nothing, or lie and say everything's fine.

What people fail to grasp is that all I really need is to be told. I have a brain that can process things logically, but before I can logically process information, that information must first be given to me. If I'm unable to gather that information on my own, I need an outside force to relay it to me.

Data and I even experience putdowns the same way.

In another episode, he's pitted in a game called Strategema against the greatest player in the Federation. Everyone concludes that because Data is a robot he cannot lose. When he does lose, everyone is disappointed and frustrated with him. People put him down: "How could you lose? How can that be?" It's easy to think that because he's a robot he won't suffer emotional trauma from putdowns. After all, he doesn't process emotions.

We later find Data in solitary confinement, replaying the game in his mind, trying to find the flaw in his tactics and discover what he did wrong and what he should have done differently. Sound familiar? Thing is, Data could find no flaw in his strategy.

Using logic to process what had happened, Data logically concluded that he was faulty, that his ability to detect fault was also faulty, and that he was therefore unfit to serve on the *Enterprise*. In fact, even when his captain needed him, Data refused to offer his service, "advising" the captain that since he was faulty he was unreliable and should not be depended on to offer any further service.

That's so often how I feel! Why is it that I set myself on a standard so much higher than anybody else? Why is it that I can give so much grace to others when they fall but whenever I make the smallest mistake I conclude that I'm unfit to serve? I've seen God take people who are alcoholic, junkies, suicidal, disabled, dying, broken, and use them in such powerful ways. Why do I so often conclude that the smallest slip makes me unusable to God?

The captain eventually had a talk with Data to encourage him into service again. I actually think the captain went about it the wrong way, though in the story his talk still worked. What he said was, "It is possible to make no mistake and still lose," which is true. What I would have said was, "It doesn't matter if you have a few glitches—you're still the best tactician on the ship and I need you."

In another episode, Data and the captain take a long elevator ride together, and out of nowhere Data starts commenting on random, distant things. When questioned about it, he answers, "I'm attempting to fill a silent moment with non-relevant conversation."

Sometimes a person will ask me a question and I'll say, "I don't have an answer yet, but I'll look it up." In other words, "Accessing…"

Right now, my family and I are watching *Terminator: The Sarah Connor Chronicles*, and I'm seeing much of my personality even in Cameron, the reformed female Terminator who the Resistance sent back in time to protect John Connor.

In one episode, the heroes are all in a facility under the guise of janitors. As Cameron mops contentedly away, awaiting further orders, Sarah runs up to her yelling that there's an enemy Terminator in the building.

Cameron continues to mop.

Sarah yells at her again, panicking.

Cameron interrupts her: "I'm thinking about what to do."

I can't keep track of the number of times a person has said something to me and been offended because I didn't respond right away. Most of the time I'm still processing what they've said, and thinking of a reply.

Honestly, there have been times when someone has asked me a question and I got up and left the room without comment—because I knew the answer was in a book in another room. I'd come back ten minutes later, give them the answer, and sit back down as if I'd been with them the whole time.

I don't get along well with fast-paced people. They tend to get impatient if I don't reply right away. If I pause between sentences, they assume I've finished talking. I even struggle talking to my pastor for this reason. He is a ridiculously fast-paced individual!

I've learned that it's nobody's fault that I struggle with fast people; we're all the way God made us. I don't feel it necessary to keep my mouth busy when I have nothing significant to say. Other people do, and that's fine. I prefer to think about my words before I speak them.

There's a guy I know who actually talks at my speed. I asked him, "Do you have Asperger's? Because you talk at the same speed I do and I have Asperger's."

I think he wasn't sure whether or not to be offended. I've had that effect on him numerous times. He simply told me, "I just think more carefully about my words before I open my mouth."

Another feature of Cameron from *The Sarah Connor Chronicles* is that she also has the ability to repeat something she's heard a person say, as if by playback from a recording device. Just like echolalia. In one episode, John, Sarah, and Cameron all have psychiatric evaluations and Cameron was diagnosed with Asperger's. My family and I burst out laughing. I now have official, psychiatric confirmation that talking to me is like talking to a robot!

A couple of people have also compared me to the character of Sheldon from *The Big Bang Theory*. I'd like to think I'm not that big a jerk, though I do see the similarities.

CHAPTER TEN

Healing Night

I f there was a cure for autism, would I take it? The question has been raised more than once over the course of my life, and the answer is always no. God intended this for me for a reason, and I wouldn't go against that. It isn't something I need to be "cured" of. Besides, I've gotten used to it, even proud of it. It's the thing that makes me unique. What would I be without it?

When taking the Alpha course for the second time, partway through my first reading of *The Purpose Driven Life* by Rick Warren, I lay praying in my cabin bed. God was up to something. I felt He was turning me to clay and preparing me to be molded. I had an unusual feeling of being exposed, bare, like a lobster that's just grown out of its cramped, hard shell.

I felt like something had left me and something else was trying to takes its place. On one hand I was glad, because although I felt vulnerable I knew it was God at work, but at the same time I felt vulnerable to attack. I spent a lot of time praying for protection for as long as I was in that state.

Two things happened over the course of the next two weeks. One, I once again considered whether or not I would take a cure for autism if one was available. And two, I prepared for the upcoming session called "Does God Heal Today?" Although there was no known scientific cure for autism, I knew it wasn't outside God's power to remove my autism if it was His will.

I again answered no, very proudly. Then I got an unexpected sense that I was hindering some of the work God was trying to do in me. I gave it some thought, took it to Him in prayer, and then realized why I was being so adamant.

I came to realize that I was relying on autism for my sense of identity (see the appendix, "Wolverine Complex"), and I was afraid of how things might change—how *I* might change, if that was taken away. I wondered if there was something God wanted me to do with my life that autism was hindering me from doing. Had the purpose of my autism reached its fulfillment? I was already aware that this was a time of change for me, and the changes already happening in my life were scary enough. I prayed on it further and asked for confirmation.

There was a rescheduling, and the Healing Night ended up taking place one week after it was previously expected. *The Purpose Driven Life*, which I had started reading on Easter, is a book that takes precisely forty days to get through. With the rescheduling, my fortieth day fell on Healing Night—which also happened to be National Prayer Day.

My center-of-the-universe mentality kicked in.

I decided to go forward for prayer, making sure that people prayed for my healing from autism *only* if it was God's will, not my will or anybody else's. If I were to be healed, then God would be praised! If I were not healed, then I would know for certain that God wanted me to use my autism as a part of my ministry, and God would still be praised! But I had to take the plunge, if only to know that I had offered everything I knew about myself as a living sacrifice to God, to do with as He saw fit.

As people prayed for me, a feeling of warmth spread through my body. My mother was there, and so was my friend Shanks. I asked them to be with me for this. As the Alpha leader prayed for me, there was an acknowledgement of some of the pain in my life, which brought me to tears. No specific events were mentioned. Perhaps the leader wasn't given specific events, or she didn't think they should be mentioned. It didn't matter which. I think I had just been trying to ignore, as hard as I could, all the pain I'd had in my life. Being permitted to acknowledge and mourn that there had been pain caused the tears.

AFTER HEALING NIGHT

My life since Healing Night has been interesting. The autism has not left me, not completely; however, some disabling aspects of it have been lifted. I have been steadily growing socially and independently. I no longer have a reason to worry about my autism being a setback. I trust that God is allowing it for His will to be fulfilled, and that He trusts me to work with it.

My friends and family tell me now that I have become more empathetic and expressive. I have apparently started using my eyebrows. I'm more adventurous and a bit more willing to socialize. I also find it easier to accept myself as I am in a social environment, and to find ways of relating to people.

There have also been some unexpected side effects. I realized sometime in my teen years that I couldn't think of my mother as anything other than something fulfilling the role of "mother." I had a hard time perceiving her as a person. This changed after Healing Night, when she finally felt an assurance in her soul that I was going to be alright, when she knew she could step away from her maternal duty and just be a friend.

It was in this time that the personality I always suspected was there but never saw finally came out. She seemed to become younger as well, and I found I could relate to her much better as a person. Before that, she hadn't let her personality shine much, which I think is part of the reason it was hard for me to separate her from "something that fulfilled the role of mother." Even though I was consciously aware of my perception of her, I didn't know what to do about it. I couldn't think of anything I *could* do. I wanted her to show me her real self, but she wouldn't. I'm glad now that I can finally have her as a friend as well.

It used to be that I could spend entire days in solitude with no social problems. As long as I knew how to feed myself breakfast and lunch (and somebody made me something healthy for dinner), I could spend entire days without having a real conversation with anyone. It's not like that anymore. Since Healing Night, I've developed a need to communicate with people. Before it was just something I could do or not do; I was okay either way. Now it's something I need on a daily basis to carry me through. I need to talk about my problems now, my worries, my fears. I need second opinions.

I need to know that I'm giving of myself for the sake of another, and that others are willing to do the same for me.

There have been some unfortunate side effects as well. About a year after Healing Night, I noticed I was becoming more aware of other people's negative social tendencies, such as hypocrisy and superficiality. This awareness seemed both familiar and forgotten, as if I'd been aware of these things as a child and trained myself to become ignorant of them. Perhaps I couldn't handle the mind games, or I didn't want to know what people were really like, or I didn't want to get caught up in it myself.

It's like what is already known because of body language has to be buried under a layer of superficial words, only the layer is a lot thinner than people pretend it is. Nothing is really hidden; we are simply expected to go along with the act and pretend our motives are more hidden than they really are.

This awareness was very uncomfortable and scary, and at first I worried that it would become a hindrance to my development. I did learn to cope with it, but it's still uncomfortable with certain groups of people. As before, I do best around people who aren't as prone to superficiality, who are comfortable with my openness and honesty.

Some of my behaviors are still distinctly Autism Spectrum. It still seems to me that the condition suits my personality. Perhaps that is why the removal has only been partial. There was only so much that I actually needed *healing* from. The rest is meant to be. If you asked my friends and family how I've changed since Healing Night, they wouldn't say I'm a different person. They would say they are able to see more of me than they could before. That's been my experience overall. I am still very much myself, just out of my shell more often.

CONCLUSION

I hope this has been helpful for anyone working to understand the autistic condition. I also hope it's been a blessing for anyone who has a heart for other people's stories. It has certainly been a joy to write.

I want to note that writing down my own history, however painful, has proved to be very therapeutic. Stuck in the moment, it's easy to feel as though I've done something wrong and that whatever happened was my fault. Being able to look at the events in hindsight (or, as I've started calling it, "God's perspective") and from a more objective viewpoint, it's easy to see how wrong it has been for people to treat me the way they did, and to see how those negative actions affected me.

Even if you have no intentions of publishing a book, I would recommend at least writing your story down. It may clear up some things.

If you'd like to read more from me and gain further insights on A.S.D., I invite you to follow my blog at benjaminfrog.wordpress.com.

I'd like to end with a verse from one of my favourite hymns:

> Before the throne of God above,
> I have a strong and perfect plea,
> A great high priest whose name is Love,
> Who ever lives and pleads for me.

My name is graven on His hands,
My name is written on His heart.
I know that while in heaven He stands,
No tongue can bid me thence depart.

The Wolverine Complex

Wolverine is a Marvel Comics superhero who is best known for his adamantium claws. His alter-ego is Logan and he's one of the X-Men. He's probably the most popular character in the whole Marvel universe next to Spider-Man.

I myself have been a fan of his from time to time—but something about him always bothered me. I noticed a recurring theme with this character that doesn't add up. Whether in comics, movies, or TV, he's always advertising. He's always using his claws, even when he's not fighting. He finds any and every excuse to bring his claws out, even in conversation. You can hardly talk to the guy without him bringing up his claws. It's as if he's afraid that if he doesn't constantly remind you of their existence, you'll forget he has them.

I wondered why this was, because Logan doesn't seem like the kind of guy who would need to do that. And then it hit me—identity.

Everyone needs an identity. Many of us don't know ourselves well enough to say who we are, so we look for other sources of identity like our possessions, our relationships, or our occupations. Logan finds his identity in his claws. He feels that he needs his claws in order to be somebody, and without them he loses his sense of self.

This is actually quite common among superheroes, so I'm not singling him out. Wolverine, however, is unique in that he actually has multiple powers. Nonetheless, he only talks about the one.

The adamantium claws were forced upon him in a horrible, unnatural, and excruciating experiment. Most people don't realize that he also has a super-human sense of smell, extreme stamina to the point that he's never fatigued, and perhaps most importantly, instantaneous healing—gifts he's had since before he can remember. But he never talks about them. There is a debate as to whether he had claws of bone before the experiment, and then had them coated in adamantium, but whenever he talks about his claws he is specifically proud of the unnatural steel.

All he wants to be known for is the adamantium claws. And if you ask people what his powers are, most of them will only talk about his claws. The majority aren't even aware of his natural gift of healing!

Every other gift he was born with, a part of who he was naturally. The adamantium claws, however, were forced onto him by scientists. They're unnatural. But Logan is unable to psychologically separate who he is naturally from what he has become through unnatural interference.

In summary, he's more proud of the unnatural part of him than all of his other natural gifts combined, finding his identity in that alone. If that unnatural thing were ever taken away, he would sooner lose his identity completely than embrace his true power.

That is what I call the Wolverine Complex.

BOOK RECOMMENDATIONS

Donna Williams, *Nobody Nowhere* (New York, NY: Doubleday, 1992).

A first-person perspective on autism. This book was a big help to me personally, as she remembers many of the aspects of severe autism I'd forgotten. She finds a way of describing it that makes you understand. It should be noted that she was diagnosed with autism, whereas I was diagnosed with Asperger's. However, the similarities between us are notable. I became high-functioning earlier in life than she did, which may be why her descriptions of severe autism are so fresh.

John Eldredge, *Wild at Heart* (Nashville, TN: Tennessee, 2001).

A good book for understanding guys in general. As someone who was never properly initiated and who never felt a connection with other guys growing up, this book was of paramount importance to me in my quest to become a man of God. It's highly unorthodox and requires a level of discretion to read. It'll throw your understanding of the world through a loop, but you'll come out of it with some relevant scriptural truths that more of the world needs to know about.

Rick Warren, *The Purpose Driven Life* (Grand Rapids, MI: Zondervan, 2002)

The Purpose Driven Life will put everything in perspective for you, not only because of what is hard to grasp on our own but also because of what is blatantly obvious that we fail to realize. I have read it three times already. It's a good get-you-back-on-the-right-track book.

Erik Rees, *S.H.A.P.E.: Finding & Fulfilling Your Unique Purpose for Life* (Grand Rapids, MI: Zondervan, 2006).

S.H.A.P.E. is an appropriate follow-up, as it shows us how to examine the unique way we've been designed by God, and how He wants to use us. I highly recommend that you read *The Purpose Driven Life* first.

The Bible.

The Bible is regarded by Christians as being the divine Word of God. It's His love letter to humanity, so it contains pretty much everything He wants to say to you. It's divided into smaller books and each one has its purpose. Out of the four Gospels, I think the book of John is the most appropriate for people who are unfamiliar with Jesus and want to know what He's about. Genesis goes over how everything got started. Psalms is a book of inspirational poems. Proverbs is a collection of wise sayings. Ecclesiastes is the personal journal of the world's wisest man while in the midst of deep depression. Judges is a book of heroes and warriors. Esther is the ultimate "comeuppance" book. Song of Songs is a book for lovers. Revelation is about the end of the world (for all you disaster lovers out there). And all the books from Romans to Jude are about the Christian life. Not to mention all the other books…

Benjamin T. Collier, *The Kingdom* (Winnipeg, MB: Word Alive Press, 2011).

There are two reasons I want to promote this book. For one, I wrote it and I get a percentage of the royalties. Two, I wrote this short novel with the intent of providing readers with a different perspective on a number of issues, including perfectionism and relationships. Some of the subject matter is mature, so I warn people not to give it to their kids, unless they've read it themselves and believe their child is mature enough for it, but I did write it with adults in mind. If you've appreciated any of the candour in the book you're reading now, you'll likely appreciate *The Kingdom* as well.

CPSIA information can be obtained at www.ICGtesting.com
Printed in the USA
LVOW11s0055140416

483457LV00008B/706/P